ABDOMINAL TRAINING

A Progressive Guide to Greater Strength

D0981255

Also available from The Lyons Press

Swimming for Fitness,
Kelvin Juba
ISBN 1-58574-550-2

The Sports Injury Handbook
Hans Kraus, M.D.
ISBN 1-5857-317-8

Marathoning A to Z
Hal Higdon
ISBN 1-58574-453-0

The Essential Swimmer
Steve Tarpanian
ISBN 1-55821-386-4

ABDOMINAL
TRAINING

A Progressive Guide to Greater Strength

CHRISTOPHER M. NORRIS

Second Edition

THE LYONS PRESS
GUILFORD, CONNECTICUT
AN IMPRINT OF THE GLOBE-PEQUOT PRESS

For Hildegard and Sophie

Copyright © 1997, 2001, 2002 by Christopher M. Norris
Published in Great Britain by A & C Black Publishers Ltd.
ISBN 1-58574-715-7
ALL RIGHTS RESERVED. No part of this book may be reproduced or
transmitted in any form by any means, electronic or mechanical, including
photocopying and recording, or by any information storage and retrieval
system, except as may be expressly permitted by the 1976 Copyright Act or
in writing from the publisher. Requests for permission should be addressed
to The Globe Pequot Press, P.O. Box 480, Guilford, CT 06437.

10 9 8 7 6 5 4 3 2 1

Printed in the United States of America
Library of Congress Cataloging-in-Publication Data is available on file.

NOTE: While very effort has been made to ensure that the content of this
book is as technically accurate and as sound as possible, neither the author
nor the publisher can accept responsibility for any injury or loss sustained
as a result of the use of this material.

Line diagrams by Jean Ashley
Figures 51 and 52 reproduced with the author's permission from Norris,
C.M. (2000) *Back Stability* (Human Kinetics, Champaign, Illinois)

CONTENTS

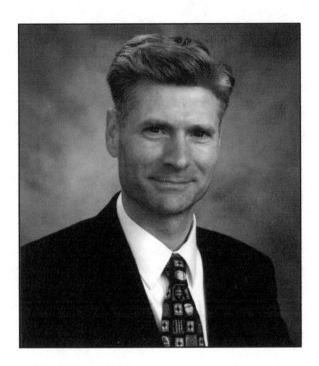

Christopher M. Norris is a licensed physiotherapist and sports scientist, an established lecturer and author of *The Complete Guide to Stretching*.

Preface

TO THE SECOND EDITION

The first edition of *Abdominal Training* has proved immensely popular both with therapists and users themselves. For the Second Edition, I have updated the text with a slightly greater emphasis on 'core stability' and placed additional exercises in each of the various sections. The concept of core stability is covered and several important exercises are included in the foundation components of the book and Levels 1–3.

In addition, there is a new chapter providing a range of case studies and sample programmes to demonstrate how you can put the various exercises in the book together in practice. On top of this, there is an important new chapter on abdominal training research. This section highlights the scientific basis of abdominal training and proves that the methods used in this book really do work. The chapter covering exercise in water has also been extended.

The results I hope will give the user a more thorough understanding of the use of functional abdominal training to enhance core stability.

Christopher M. Norris

INTRODUCTION

There are many types of training available today, each with a specific aim. Some aim to reduce weight, others to strengthen muscle, and still others to increase general fitness. Most fashionable abdominal exercise programmes are designed to work the mid-section hard and make the muscles 'hurt', in the belief that this will 'flatten the tummy' or 'trim the waist'. They are normally based on exercise to music classes, or on sport. These programmes often talk about 'going for the burn' and 'pumping up'. Unfortunately, they are not suitable for those of poor or even average fitness levels, firstly because they are too demanding, and secondly because they place excessive stress on the lower back.

The abdominal programme described in this book is very different. It does not come from a sporting background, but from physiotherapy exercises designed to rehabilitate the spine following injury. As such it aims to be both safe and effective, and to develop trunk fitness which is relevant to everyday life rather than just to sport. In physiotherapy terms, this type of training is called 'functional', hence the term Functional Load Abdominal Training (F.L.A.T.).

HOW THE SPINE WORKS

OVERVIEW OF THE SPINAL COLUMN

The human backbone, or 'spinal column', is made up of 33 bones. Each bone is called a 'vertebra', and the vertebrae are formed into five groups (*see* fig. 1). In the neck the bones, called 'cervical vertebrae', are delicate but highly mobile, enabling you to turn your head fully. In the chest region the bones are called 'thoracic vertebrae' and these bones connect to the ribs. In the lower spine the spinal bones are called 'lumbar vertebrae'. These are large, strong bones covered with powerful muscles. Below the lumbar vertebrae are the remnants of our tail. The 'sacrum' is a triangular shaped bone which attaches at the sides to the pelvis, while the 'coccyx' forms a thin, pointed tip to the end of the spine.

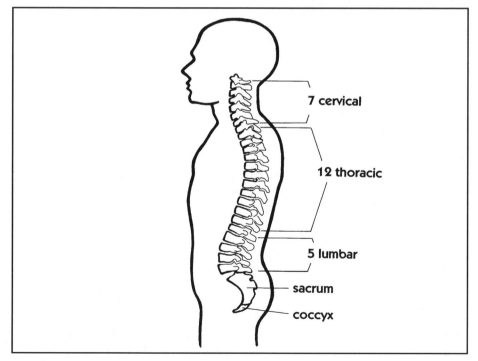

Fig. 1 *The spinal column*

SPINAL CURVES •

Although the spinal vertebrae stand one on top of each other, the column they make is not straight. Instead, the spine forms an 'S' curve. There are two inward curves in the lower back and neck, while the thoracic spine curves gently outwards. These curves are not present at birth, but begin to develop in early childhood.

In the early years of life, a baby's spine is rounded, and we call this rounded shape the 'primary spinal curve' (*see* fig. 2a). As the baby starts to lie on its front and lift its head up, the neck curve starts to form (*see* fig. 2b). It is not until a baby stands up that the curve in the lower back is formed (*see* fig. 2c). Because the neck and lower back curves form later, they are called 'secondary spinal curves'.

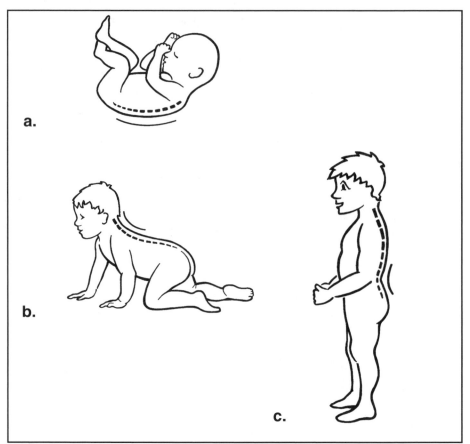

Fig. 2 *(a) Primary spinal curve; (b) secondary curve in neck; (c) secondary curve in lower back*

If the spine was completely straight, when we run or jump a large amount of shock would be transmitted up to the head. The function of the spinal curves is to enable the spine to act in a spring-like fashion, absorbing some of the shock of movement and making actions more agile.

When the spinal curves are altered, stress can be placed on the spine. This can occur through alterations in posture and the way we work. Long periods spent sitting at desks and driving a car will change the important curve in the lumbar region and this can be one source of low back pain.

• • • • • • • • • • • • • • • *KEYPOINT* • • • • • • • • • • • • • • • • •
Maintaining a correct curve in the lower back is important to overall spinal health.

THE SPINAL SEGMENT •

Each pair of spinal bones together forms a single unit called a 'spinal segment' (*see* fig. 3). The two bones are separated by a spongy disc attached to the flat part of the bone. At the back of the vertebra the bone is extended to form two small joints called 'facets'. From above it can be seen that the back of the spinal bone forms a hollow arch through which runs the spinal cord carrying messages from the brain to the legs and arms (*see* fig. 4).

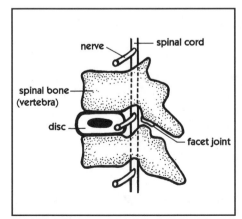

Fig. 3 *The spinal segment*

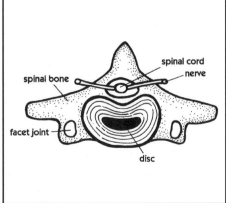

Fig. 4 *Cross section through the spine*

SPINAL LIGAMENTS

Bending forwards will stretch the ligaments behind the spine but relax those in front. Bending backwards will reverse the situation, stretching the front ligaments but relaxing those covering the back of the spine. If you perform an exercise which persistently overstretches a ligament, the ligament will become sore and inflamed. This may take time to develop, so you may not feel pain at the time. Instead, you frequently have back ache the next day. If this is the case, change your exercise programme.

If a bent position of the spine is held regularly, perhaps as part of your job, overstretched ligaments will lengthen and those which are relaxed will shorten markedly. This is what happens with poor posture (*see* pages 37–49). If you are the sort of person who spends most of their day slumped in a chair, your spinal ligaments will alter, making it harder for you to hold your spine in a correct alignment when you stand up. To correct this, you must practise exercises to correct your spinal alignment and try to correct your general posture throughout the day.

> **•••••••••••••••• KEYPOINT ••••••••••••••••••**
> Repeated bending movements overstretch the spine and can damage it. Cut down on your bending!

NERVES

The spinal cord consists of thousands of tiny nerve fibres bunched together much like a telephone cable. In the same way as the telephone line, the nerves carry electrical messages. When you want to move your leg, for example, an electrical message is sent from the brain. It travels down a nerve contained in your spinal cord to the muscles in your leg, commanding them to move.

A similar message can move in the opposite direction. If you touch a hot object, an electrical message is sent from your hand up a nerve in your arm through the spinal cord and to the area in your brain responsible for feeling. At any time, thousands of electrical impulses are travelling up and down the nerves in your body. If something blocks these impulses, the electrical messages change, and both movement and feeling can be affected. This is what happens when you trap a nerve. The nerve becomes compressed, a little like stepping on a hose pipe. When this happens the impulses for movement and feeling can become blocked, you get tingling sensations and numbness, and your muscles may twitch or become weak. These sensations can be felt wherever the nerve travels. Often with the lower back the feelings travel into the buttock and leg and then right down to the foot.

• • • • • • • • • • • • • • • • **KEYPOINT** • • • • • • • • • • • • • • • • •
Pain or 'strange feelings' in your leg could be caused by an injury to your back.

DISC STRUCTURE, FUNCTION AND INJURY • • • • • • • • • •

The disc is the structure which separates the bodies of the two adjacent spinal bones. The disc acts like a shock absorber, preventing the spine from being shaken or jarred when we walk and run. Each disc has a hard outer casing which contains a softer spongy gel called the 'disc nucleus' (*see* fig. 5). Importantly, this gel has no direct blood supply, but instead relies on movement for its health. As the spine moves, fluids are pressed into the disc nucleus and waste products are squeezed out, keeping the disc healthy. As we get older the disc gel begins to dry up and becomes more brittle. When this happens the spine gets stiffer, and so you are no longer able to turn the cartwheels of your youth when you retire! However, through regular exercise, the disc stays springy for longer.

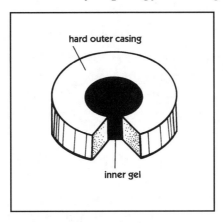

hard outer casing

inner gel

Fig. 5 *The structure of the spinal disc*

If we were to look at the discs of someone who is 30 years old but inactive, and compare them to someone who is 40 but fit, the two discs would probably be exactly the same. The discs of the fitter person have stayed younger because they have been fed through regular movement.

• • • • • • • • • • • • • • • **KEYPOINT** • • • • • • • • • • • • • • • •
The disc needs regular movement to stay healthy.

As we move the spine, the spinal bones tip forwards and backwards, and as they do so they press the discs out of shape. When this happens the gel in the disc is squeezed and its pressure increases. Because we bend forwards much more often than we bend backwards, the gel in the disc starts to move backwards towards the delicate nerves of the spine. When this happens we begin to get pain. Initially this is a dull ache which occurs only occasionally. If we continue to do too much bending, however, we will begin to feel the pain more regularly and it will be more intense as the disc gradually becomes more damaged. Eventually, after many years of repeated bending, the gel in the centre of the disc can burst out and press on to one of the delicate nerves. When this happens it is termed a 'slipped disc', a particularly painful condition.

It is important to remember that it is *repeated* bending – stressing the disc over and over again – which is the real villain here. More people suffer from back pain brought on by bending the spine, through slumping in a poor chair or stooping when they work, than from lifting a heavy weight.

• • • • • • • • • • • • • • • **KEYPOINT** • • • • • • • • • • • • • • • •
Repeated bending squeezes the discs. Over many years
damage accumulates and the discs can suddenly burst. This is
a slipped disc.

THE IMPORTANCE OF SPINAL FACET JOINTS • • • • • • • • •

The 'facets' are two small joints at the back of the vertebrae. They are similar in construction to other joints in the body in that they are contained within a tough leathery bag called a 'capsule'. As we bend forwards, the facet joint opens up, and as we bend back the joint closes. Twisting the spine results in the surfaces of the facet joint sliding over each other (*see* fig. 6).

Because these joints are so small, rapid movements can cause them to move too far and so damage them. Bending forwards repeatedly when practising stretching exercises, for example, can overstretch the leathery capsule of the facet joints, leaving the spine looser than it should be and therefore susceptible to injury. Bending backwards suddenly, as can be seen in some weight training exercises, closes the facet joints rapidly with a sudden 'jolt'. Over time this can cause premature wearing of these delicate joints.

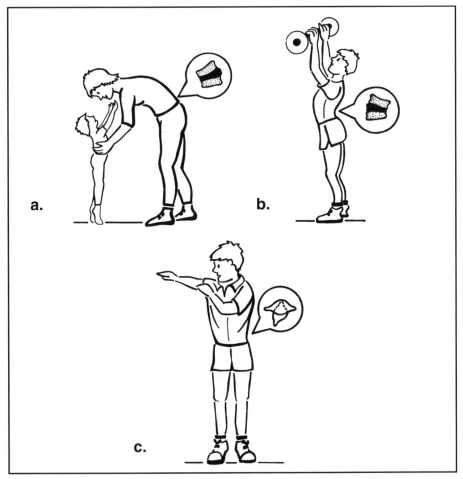

Fig. 6 *Spinal joint movement: (a) bending opens the spinal joints; (b) reaching up closes the spinal joints; (c) twisting causes the spinal joints to slide over each other*

••••••••••••••• *KEYPOINT* •••••••••••••••••
Rapid movements can jolt the small facet joints at the back of
the spine, over and over again.

RANGE OF MOVEMENT ••••••••••••••••••••••••

The total extent of movement which is possible at any joint is
called its 'range of movement'. Normally, in everyday living, we
operate with our joints moving in the middle of this range. This
is really the safest part because the joint is in no danger of being
overstretched and the muscles feel comfortable.

With each movement, damage can only occur if the joint is
pressed as far as it can go. We call this end point of movement
the 'end range'. When we are exercising, if we push our joints to
the end range over and over again we can damage them. A safer
method is to practise exercises for which the great majority of
movements are in the middle of the movement range. In this
way there is a good margin of safety (*see* fig. 7). In the F.L.A.T.
programme almost all of the exercises are performed using the
spine in the middle of its range of movement to guard against
injury.

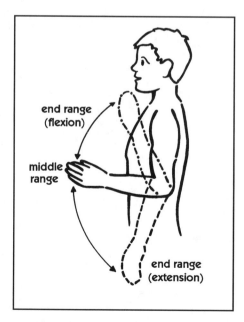

end range
(flexion)

middle
range

end range
(extension)

Fig. 7 *Range of movement*

●●●●●●●●●●●●●●●● ***KEYPOINT*** ●●●●●●●●●●●●●●●●●
Exercises which use the middle part of a joint's movement are safer than those which take the joint to the end point of its movement.

LUMBAR AND PELVIC MOVEMENTS ● ● ● ● ● ● ● ● ● ● ● ● ● ●

Excessive movement in the lumbar spine can occur without us noticing it. If a person bends forwards to touch their toes or backwards to look at the ceiling, the movement is obvious. But there is another way that the lumbar spine can move which is more subtle.

The pelvis is connected directly to the lumbar spine (*see* fig. 8) and in turn balances rather like a seesaw on the hip joints. Because it is balanced, the pelvis can tilt forwards and backwards. As it tilts, the pelvis pulls the spine with it. If the pelvis tips down (*see* fig. 8a) the arch in the lumbar spine increases in a way equivalent to moving the spine backwards into 'extension'. When the pelvis tilts up (*see* fig. 8c) the lumbar curve is flattened, and the movement in the lumbar spine is equivalent to 'flexion', or forward bending.

If the movement of the pelvis is excessive, the spine in turn is pulled to its end range, stressing the spinal tissues. Note that it is only the lumbar spine which is moving. The rest of the spine remains largely unchanged, so the person is still standing upright.

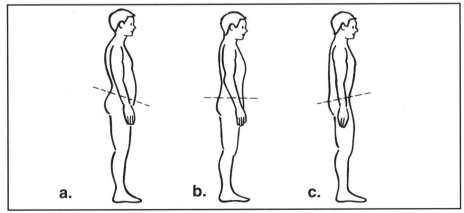

Fig. 8 *Pelvic movement: (a) forward tilting – lower back hollow; (b) normal – lower back neutral; (c) backward tilting – lower back flattens*

• • • • • • • • • • • • • • • • • *KEYPOINT* • • • • • • • • • • • • • • • • • •
Movement of the pelvis directly affects the lumbar spine.

THE NEUTRAL POSITION OF THE LUMBAR SPINE • • • • • • •

We have seen that as we move the spine the alignment of the spinal bones and tissues change. For example, as we flex forwards the facet joints open and the tissues on the back of the spine stretch while those on the front relax. At the same time the pressure within the spinal discs increases. This combination of pressure and stretch, if repeated over and over again, can damage the spinal tissues.

If, however, we align the spinal tissues so the spine is upright and the lumbar region is comfortably curved, the spinal tissues are now at their normal length and the pressure within the discs is lowered. We call this normal alignment of the spine the 'neutral position' (*see* fig. 8b). It is one of the safest postures for the spine, so all the elementary F.L.A.T. exercises begin with the spine in the neutral position.

To find your own neutral position, stand with your back to a wall. Your buttocks and shoulders should touch the wall. Place the flat of your hand between the wall and the small of your back. Try to tilt your pelvis so you flatten your back and then tilt your pelvis the other way so you increase the hollow in the lower back. Your neutral position (and it is slightly different for each person) is halfway between the flat and hollow positions.

You should just be able to place the flat of your hand between your back and the wall. If you can only place your fingers through, your back is too flat; if your whole hand up to your wrist can pass through the space, your back is too hollow (*see* page 42).

(*see* page 42)

• • • • • • • • • • • • • • • • *KEYPOINT* • • • • • • • • • • • • • • • • • • •
In the neutral position the spine is correctly aligned and the spinal tissues are held at the right length.

CORE STABILITY ●

If we can maintain the neutral position of the spine when we move or lift, for example, we can greatly reduce the stress on the spinal tissues. This is an essential part of the concept of core stability. In simple terms, core stability literally means holding the centre part of the body firm so that the limbs (arms and legs) will have a stable base upon which to move. The concept of holding one part firm so that another part can move effectively is not new, of course, and is seen in all sorts of common daily activities. When we drive a car, for example, we put our foot on the accelerator and expect the car to go forward. For this to happen, the tyre must grip on the road surface and the road must stay firm or 'stable'. If the tyre grips on ice instead, the wheel simply spins and forward movement of the car cannot occur.

INTERACTING COMPONENTS OF STABILITY ● ● ● ● ● ● ● ● ● ●

The core of the body is the part between the pelvis and the ribcage, and this relies on muscle to hold it firm. Core stability results from the interplay between three body components (*see* fig. 9). The first is the shape of the bones and joints. This is called the 'passive' component because it is moved by muscles or forces *outside* the body, such as heavy weight, but is not able to move by itself. If the passive system breaks down, the body core will loose stability. A broken bone, or dislocated joint, for example, will leave the body virtually unable to move because the bodypart is insecure. No matter how much we pull or push on it, the pain and

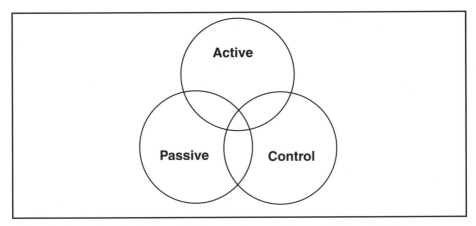

Fig. 9 *Interplay between body components providing stability*

instability will stop us moving effectively. The body quite rightly recognises that this will damage us and forces us to rest.

The next component which contributes to core stability is the 'active' system. This is made up of the muscles which pull on the bones and joints either to hold them firm or to move them. In order to do this effectively, the muscles must be sufficiently strong. Using the example of the broken bone above, if we place the limb in a plaster cast the bone will heal: the 'passive' system (bone) therefore becomes more solid or 'stable'. However, when we remove the plaster cast all the muscles will have wasted and we are both too weak to move the limb very far, and too weak to hold it firm (stable). This is why after a fracture the leg often 'gives way' when we twist or turn suddenly. The passive stability (bones) is fine, but the active stability (muscle) is weak.

When the muscles become strong, we cannot use them all the time because they will get tired, and we do not want tense muscles continually. The ideal situation is to be able to turn the muscles on and off so that we can use them to stabilise the body when we need them to and allow them to rest when we don't. Economy of movement is the key here, and this is the job of the third stability component, 'control'. This system works by the brain and spinal cord monitoring tiny sensors in the joints and muscles of the body. These sensors give us information about body position, movement, and stress and strain which is imposed on the body through everyday activities. When a joint or bodypart is put under strain, the sensors will detect this and send a message to the muscles to tighten and hold that part of the body firm – or 'stabilise' it – to resist the forces stressing it.

This process of force detection and muscle reaction is the job of the control system. In some people this is very good and runs extremely smoothly. In a ballet dancer, for example, the muscles may be small and lean, but because the body control is very good the dancer can use just the right amount of muscle force to hold the body stable and control each action with great precision. After a knee injury, a rugby player may still have much bigger muscles than the ballet dancer, but through pain the body control has been lost. The muscles shake and quiver as the knee is moved and the actions are ungainly and poorly controlled.

In the case of the lumbar spine, which is clearly in the centre of the body, the stability provided by the active, passive and control systems is of the 'core' or the body. In this case the active system is that of the abdominal and lumbar muscles (*see* pages 15–17), while the passive system consists of the spinal bones, discs and ligaments. The control system integrating these two comes from nervous impulses in both the spine and brain. The muscles of the active sub-system can be divided into the surface (superficial) muscles of the rectus abdominis and the external obliques which primarily move the core region, and the deeper muscles, transversus abdominis and internal obliques which mainly *prevent excessive movement* of the body core and 'stabilise' it.

Thus, for effective core stability, a subtle interplay between the three stability systems is required. The bones and joints must move freely, the muscles must be strong and supple, and the body control must be well coordinated. Failure of any one of these systems will reduce core stability. Importantly, however, if this does occur, correctly applied exercise can often build up the other two stability components to compensate. Take arthritis as an example. In this condition there is wear and tear of the joints. This can often leave the joint less stable with a tendency to give way. In this situation, a physiotherapist can give a patient special exercises to strengthen the muscles which support the joint and improve the body control by using skilled movements. The *active* and *control* components of stability are therefore built up to compensate for the *passive* system which is worn. Although the bones cannot be changed, the patient enjoys virtually full, pain-free actions because the body has compensated for the damaged joints and bones.

LOCAL AND GLOBAL MUSCLES

We have two sets of muscles contributing to core stability (*see* page 16). Some are close to the central core of the body and are called 'local' muscles. Others are quite far away from the central core and are called 'global' muscles. The *local* muscles, close to the spine and pelvis, act to move the spine subtly and adjust it with fine movements to keep the posture correct and make sure the body alignment is optimal. The *global* muscles, on the other hand, do not make fine adjustments of spinal position, but instead take some of the strain which the body is subjected to before this strain can damage the spine. When lifting, for example, the large leg muscles (global) can be used to provide the power for the lift while the deep muscle corset (local) can maintain the neutral position of the lower spine.

Often, after a bout of back pain, the local muscles are turned off and quickly waste (become lax). When we move, we loose subtle movements of the spine and rely instead on our large global muscles. Our movements become clumsy and poorly coordinated, and the muscles often become tight, tense and painful. Our backs feel stiff after a bout of gardening, for example, and the muscles feel tight and cord-like. Instead of using the subtle local musculature of the body core, we have used the strong global muscles. They are too powerful for this task, however, and quickly go into spasm, giving pain. If we make the mistake of trying to strengthen the back in a gym using heavy weight training techniques, these already firm global muscles can be built up even further without the subtle local muscles being worked, so we end up with an imbalance between the two sets of muscles resulting in further pain.

The gentle foundation movements given in this book are designed to restore muscle balance, and work to improve core stability because they target the *local* muscles. Once these have been performed and core stability has been improved, the exercises gradually bring in the *global* muscles to build complete 'spinal fitness'.

SUMMARY

- The spine is divided into regions: *cervical* (neck), *thoracic* (rib cage), *lumbar* (lower back), *sacrum* and *coccyx* (tailbone) (*see* page 1).
- The spine forms an 'S' curve, making it naturally springy.
- Bending and straightening the spine stretches and relaxes the spinal ligaments.
- Nerves transmit electrical messages for movement and feeling.
- If a nerve is trapped, movement and feeling can alter, giving weakness, pain or tingling.
- The disc contains a gel and acts as a shock-absorber.
- Safe movement keeps the discs healthy, but poor movements allow stress to build in the discs over many years.
- Mid-range is the centre part of the total extent of movement possible at a joint.
- In its neutral position, the spine is correctly aligned and the spinal tissues are at their normal length.
- Back stability depends on the interaction between the *passive* (bones), *active* (muscle) and *control* (coordination) components of the body.
- Muscles *local* to the spine control the subtle position of the spinal bones. Muscles some distance away from the spine (*global*) help to minimise forces before they can reach the spine.

THE TRUNK MUSCLES

The muscles which concern us in the F.L.A.T. programme are those which are arranged around the trunk. At the front and sides are the four principal abdominal muscles, at the back the spinal extensors and multifidus, and at the base of the trunk the pelvic floor muscle.

In the centre of the abdomen is the 'rectus abdominis'. This muscle runs from the lower ribs to the pubic region, forming a narrow strap. It tapers down from about 15 cm (6 in.) wide at the top to 8 cm (3 in.) wide at the bottom. The muscle has three fibrous bands across it at the level of the tummy button, and above and below this point (*see* fig. 10a). The rectus muscle on each side of the body is contained within a sheath, the two sheaths merging in the centre line of the body via a strong fibrous band. This region splits during pregnancy to allow for the bulk of the developing child.

At the side of the abdomen there are two diagonal muscles, the 'internal oblique' (*see* fig. 10e) and the 'external oblique' (*see* fig. 10d). The internal oblique attaches to the front of the pelvic bone and a strong ligament in this region. From here it travels up and across to the lower ribs and into the sheath covering the rectus muscle. The external oblique has a similar position, but lies at an angle to the internal oblique. The external oblique begins from the lower eight ribs and travels to the sheath covering the rectus muscle and to the strong pelvic ligaments. The fibres in the centre of the muscle are travelling diagonally, but those right on the edge are travelling vertically and will assist the rectus muscle in its action.

Underneath the oblique abdominals lies the 'transversus abdominis'. This attaches from the pelvic bones and tissue covering the spinal muscles and travels horizontally forwards to merge with the sheath covering the rectus muscle (*see* fig. 10c). At the side and back of the trunk, the 'quadratus lumborum' muscle is also important (*see* fig. 10f). It is positioned between the pelvis and rib cage, and has an inner and outer portion. When we are performing abdominal exercises to enhance core stability we must also be aware of the 'pelvic floor' muscles. These attach to the inside of the pelvis and form a sort of sling running from the tailbone (coccyx) at the back to the pubic bone (crotch) at the front. The muscles from each side of the body join in the middle, and the front and back passages (vagina, urethra

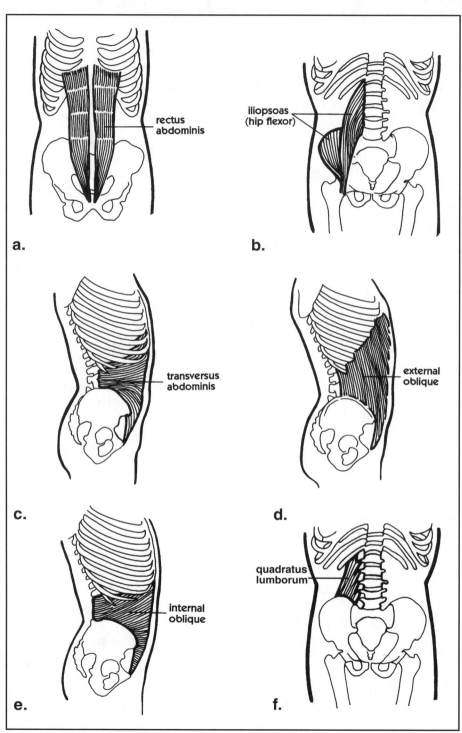

Fig. 10 *The abdominal and hip flexor muscles*

and anus) are formed within the pelvic floor muscles. These openings are controlled by rings of muscle called 'sphincters' which lie in the pelvic floor.

All these muscles work together, and so in any action involving the abdomen, most of the muscles will be active to a certain extent. In a sit-up action, the upper portion of the rectus is emphasised, while in pelvic tilting the lower portion of this muscle and the outer fibres of the external oblique are used more. Twisting actions involve the oblique abdominals, while the transversus acting with the obliques pulls the tummy in tight. This muscle is used in coughing and sneezing as well. Together with the obliques, the outer portion of the quadratus is important for side bending actions and also pulls on the lower ribs when breathing deeply. The inner portion is next to the spine and helps to support it in actions which tend to pull you sideways. The quadratus is therefore important to core stability when carrying an object in one hand – for example, a shopping basket or case. After pregnancy (*see* page 25), following certain types of lower back pain, and in very obese individuals, the pelvic floor muscles reduce their tone and people can sometimes loose control of the sphincters and dribble urine. For this reason, regaining control of the pelvic floor is important and can be achieved at the same time as re-educating the deep muscle corset (transversus and internal oblique). As we shall see (page 18), the pelvic floor muscles are also integral to the creation of pressure which forms the 'abdominal balloon', an important process in developing core stability.

SUMMARY

• The rectus muscle bends the trunk and lifts the tail when lying on the back.
• The obliques twist the spine.
• Transversus pulls the tummy in tight.
• The quadratus lumborum muscle stiffens the spine when a force tries to bend the spine sideways.
• The pelvic floor muscles can be re-educated at the same time as core stability.

HOW THE TRUNK MUSCLES ACT FOR CORE STABILITY ● ● ●

There are several methods by which the trunk muscles can make the trunk more solid and contribute to core stability.

THE ABDOMINAL BALLOON

If we look at the trunk (*see* fig. 11) we can imagine it as a cylinder. The walls of the cylinder are the oblique abdominal muscles which form the deep muscle corset (transversus, internal obliques and multifidus). The top of the cylinder is formed by the diaphragm, a sheet of muscle tissue which 'cuts the body in half' and is found beneath the chest and above the tummy. This muscle enables us to breathe, pulling air into the lungs and forcing it out again like a pair of bellows. When we breath in, the diaphragm goes down to pull air into the lungs. Because it goes down, the top of our 'cylinder' is squashed in, much like pressing on the top of a drinks can, for example. The floor of the cylinder is formed by the pelvic floor muscles, the ones which make us 'hold on' when we are desperate to go to the toilet but can't find the bathroom (*see* page 17)! When we do this, these muscles are pulled into the body slightly giving us the feeling that we are pulling in and upwards between the legs.

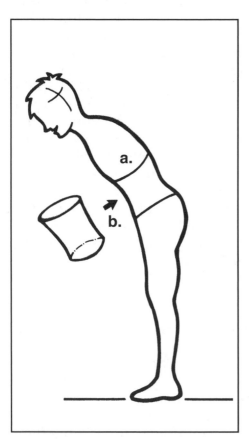

Fig. 11 The 'abdominal balloon': the diaphragm (a) moves downwards as the deep muscle corset tightens and the abdominal walls (b) are pulled in

When all three sets of muscles work together, the cylinder is squeezed in every direction: the top is pulling in, the bottom is pulling up, and the walls are squeezing inwards. Contained within the cylinder are the stomach, intestines and body organs and, as the muscles squeeze in, the whole area acts like a giant balloon, providing a solid 'bubble' at the front of the trunk. As we lift a heavy object there is a tendency for the spine to buckle and bend forwards (flex), but the abdominal balloon – positioned at the front of the body – helps to stop this happening.

Heavy lifts or rapid movements of the trunk result in stronger muscle contractions and so the pressure produced by the abdominal balloon is greater. As this pressure is within the abdomen, it is called 'Intra Abdominal Pressure', or IAP. The larger the IAP, the better a person's core stability, and this is achieved by having deep abdominal muscles which are strong, but more importantly able to hold the area firm for long periods. This is why holding, or muscle endurance, is important to core stability (*see* page 28).

Interestingly, because all three sets of muscles which form the cylinder have to tighten at the same time, the coordination of this action can break down. One example of this is the incontinence which some young mums suffer. This occurs sometimes when they cough or laugh because both of these actions increase the IAP. Although the pressure is increasing, the pelvic-floor muscles are poorly toned and poorly controlled after pregnancy and so the pressure causes urine (water) to press out of the bladder unrestrained. The answer is to restore the feeling that the muscles between the legs are pulling 'in and up' by using special pelvic-floor exercises and also targeting the deep muscle corset (*see* page 92).

• • • • • • • • • • • • • • • **KEYPOINT** • • • • • • • • • • • • • • • •
Coordination and timing between several muscles is required to create an effective abdominal balloon.

BACK FASCIA

The second method by which core stability is created involves a sheet of tough elastic material which stretches from the back of the ribcage to the pelvis. The material is called 'fascia' and because this particular piece stretches across the upper back (thoracic spine) and lower back (lumbar spine) it is called the 'Thoraco-Lumbar Fascia' or TLF. As we lift an object and are pulled forwards by its weight, the fascia is stretched. However, several muscles work to pull on the fascia and tighten it, enabling it to resist this force because:

• The transversus muscle and the internal oblique surround the trunk and attach at the back to the fascia. When they tighten they pull the fascia from the sides, similar to the effect of pulling on the side of someones shirt to flatten it.

• The back muscles (spinal extensors) are two strong vertical columns running up either side of the spine. They are encased in a layer of the fascia, and when they contract they stretch the fascia and tighten it.

• The buttock muscles (gluteals) and the muscles which pull your arms to your sides (latissimus dorsi) connect to the top and bottom of the fascia. They tighten it by pulling it upwards and downwards at the same time as the deep abdominal muscles pull it sideways.

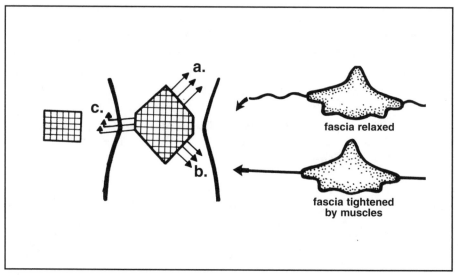

Fig. 12 *The back fascia (a) latissimus dorsi (b) gluteals (c) internal oblique, transversus*

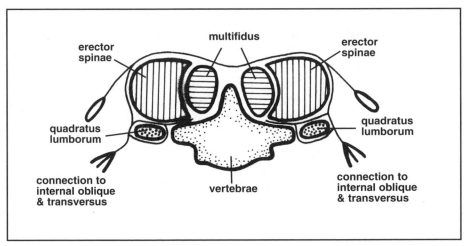

Fig. 13 *Cross-section of the trunk*

The net result of all this muscular activity is to strengthen the spine and help it resist the bending forces which are seen in lifting. They create an effective mechanism, but one which will only be able to functional optimally if the muscles are strong and able to pull for a long period of time. In addition, the muscles must work at the right time in a lift. If they pull too soon their force will do no good, and if they pull after the weight has been lifted, the stress will already have been placed on the spine. Again, coordination is important. The muscles must pull at just the right time, with just the right amount of force – and, after a bout of back pain or a long period of inactivity, this mechanism takes training and practice to restore.

BACK EXTENSOR MUSCLES

There are two groups of back extensor muscles which are important to core stability, especially in lifting. The first are local muscles (*see* pages 13–4) which attach between each of the vertebrae, and the second are global muscles (*see* pages 13–4) which attach along the whole length of the spine.

Of the local group, the 'multifidus' muscle is particularly important. This not only moves the spinal bones in relation to each other – in other words, it produces a rocking action of one bone against the other in the same way as one brick can move within a column of bricks – but also flattens the lumbar curve without moving the whole spine. Probably the most important feature of this muscle, however, is its ability to stiffen the spine. Because it is positioned between the spinal bones, it acts a little like cement between bricks. A column of bricks stacked on top of each other is very unstable. However, if the bricks are cemented together with mortar, they are very stable. Any amount of pressing and pulling will be withstood, and the column will remain standing. The multifidus has a similar function in that it stiffens the spine and helps it to resist bending forces. However, after a back injury or bout of low back pain, it becomes much smaller and weaker and so the spine is more susceptible to further injury. Unfortunately, when the back pain has been resolved, the multifidus does not build itself back up again readily. It needs to be 'reminded' how to work through the use of special exercises (*see* page 91).

The global spinal muscles are the spinal extensors which lie on either side of the spine. As we saw above, they are like two powerful columns which support the spine as we bend forwards and move the back from the vertical to a more horizontal position. Although the strength of these muscles is important, their endurance – how long they can hold themselves tight – is actually more significant. This is because if the endurance of the muscles is poor, they will gradually allow the back to slip into an increasingly poor posture after repeated bending activities. Think of the spine as a fishing rod. Instead of only heavy fish causing the rod to bend enticingly, the rod has weakened so that *any* fish caught on the line looks like a whopper! The result is the same. The rod, or in this case the spine, bends more and more. Therefore the amount of time someone can spend tightening the back muscles and holding them tight is the important factor, especially with intensive activities such as sport or heavy lifting. This is why we target these muscles with a number of exercises, ultimately leading to the spinal extension hold shown on page 124.

● ● ● ● ● ● ● ● ● ● ● ● ● ● ● **KEYPOINT** ● ● ● ● ● ● ● ● ● ● ● ● ● ● ●
The amount of time someone can tighten the back muscles and hold them tight (endurance) is more important than pure strength.

SELECTING WHICH MUSCLES TO WORK • • • • • • • • • • • •

The abdominal muscles can either be used for movement, to bend or twist the trunk, for example, or for stability. When used for stability, the muscles hold the spine firm, preventing excessive movement. In order to do this, they work to make the trunk into a more solid cylinder. For instance, when we are lifting something or pushing and pulling, the spine has to form a solid base for the arms and legs to push against. If not, the force created by the limbs will move the trunk rather than moving the object it was intended to.

Any of the trunk muscles can be activated by appropriate exercises to move the spine. However, to stabilise the spine it is the muscles deep inside the body, and therefore next to the spine, which are used. The transversus and the deep back muscles are your most important stability muscles, and they are helped by the obliques. The rectus muscle and the muscles near the surface of the back are responsible for rapid movements such as sitting up from lying, or standing up straight again from a bent over position.

• • • • • • • • • • • • • • • *KEYPOINT* • • • • • • • • • • • • • • • •
The deep trunk muscles make the spine more stable, holding the spinal bones together. The muscles on the surface cause movement.

THE HIP MUSCLES •

The major hip muscle affected during abdominal training is the 'hip flexor' ('iliopsoas'). It attaches in two parts. The first part comes from the lumbar spine, the second from the pelvis (*see* fig. 10b). Both parts merge to fasten on to the thighbone. The action of this muscle is best illustrated when lying flat on your back. If you lift one leg, the hip flexor has acted to bend the hip. If you sit up from lying flat, keeping your back straight and bending at the hip, the muscle has acted to pull your trunk up.

Because the muscle attaches to each vertebra of the lumbar spine, as it contracts it will pull the lumbar vertebrae together. As this happens the pressure within the vertebra will increase –

we have seen that increased pressure within the discs is one cause of lower back pain. For this reason all the exercises used in the F.L.A.T. programme aim to reduce the work of the hip flexor. Where this muscle is working, the lumbar spine must be kept in its neutral position.

• • • • • • • • • • • • • • • **KEYPOINT** • • • • • • • • • • • • • • • •
If the hip flexor muscle is worked too hard it will pull on the lower spine, dangerously increasing the pressure within the discs.

HOW MUSCLES CAUSE MOVEMENT • • • • • • • • • • • • • •

Muscle consists of many fibres running parallel to each other. If we look through a microscope at these fibres we see that they contain a series of interlocking finger-like projections. When a muscle contracts, the finger projections pull together and overlap, shortening the muscle. So, as a muscle contracts it will pull. This is all it can do; it cannot push. For example, if you bend your arm the muscles on the inside of the arm pull the forearm towards the upper arm. The muscles on the outside of the arm cannot push the arm into this position. They must actually relax to allow the movement to occur.

The more the finger projections within the muscle can overlap, the stronger the muscle will be. If the muscle starts from a position where the projections are already overlapped and the muscle is shortened, the force the muscle can produce is very small because there is little further movement available. If the muscle is overstretched, the finger-like projections can't overlap sufficiently and so again the muscle appears weak. For maximum strength gains then, the muscle should be contracted from a comfortable lengthened position, not too short (cramped) or overstretched.

The other function of a muscle is to act like a giant elastic band. When stretched, the tissue within the muscle will spring back, and we call this 'recoil' or 'elastic strength'. When we look at the abdominal muscles during an exercise, we must consider how each muscle is acting to create a movement, and how it could limit a movement because of its length.

• • • • • • • • • • • • • • • • *KEYPOINT* • • • • • • • • • • • • • • • • • •
A muscle can only pull; it cannot push.

ABDOMINAL MUSCLES AND PREGNANCY • • • • • • • • • • •

During pregnancy the abdominal muscles have to stretch to accommodate the growing child. The muscles are able to stretch lengthways quite substantially, but their ability to stretch sideways is limited. The sideways increase in space is brought about by splitting of the tissue which joins the two neighbouring rectus muscles in the centre line of the body (*see* fig. 14). The split is called a 'diastasis' and its size is dependent on a number of factors. Mothers who have a narrow pelvis or a large baby (over 9 lb) are likely to have a large diastasis, as are those who have twins or triplets. If a mother has been inactive during her pregnancy or has not toned up the abdominal muscles following a previous pregnancy, again the diastasis may be larger.

During pregnancy the abdominal hollowing action and pelvic tilting (*see* pages 83–6) are important to reduce the strain on the abdominal wall and the spine. Following child birth, the diastasis must be allowed to close before very active abdominal exercises are begun. Abdominal hollowing is particularly useful during the early stages (from three days following child birth). The action should be practised regularly throughout the day to

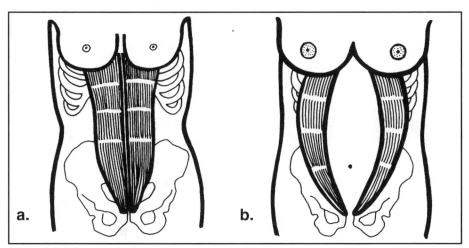

Fig. 14 *The abdominal muscles in pregnancy: (a) normal; (b) following child birth*

re-educate the abdominal muscles. It is often easier to practise this movement while breast feeding in a sitting or lying position: the young mother has little time available, and the feeding period may be the only respite she has.

Pelvic tilting is also important during the first weeks after child birth. The aim now is to correct any exaggerated 'lordosis' which occurs through a forward-tilted pelvis (*see* fig. 8a, page 9). Whenever the young mum is standing, she should try to do so without an excessive curve in the lower spine.

The oblique abdominal muscles pull on to the area of the tummy which has split during pregnancy. Forcible contraction of the obliques may therefore slow the closure of the diastasis, so twisting actions against resistance should not be practised until the diastasis has closed to a width of two fingers.

SUMMARY

• The split in the abdominal muscles which occurs during pregnancy is called a 'diastasis'.
• The diastasis may be larger if you have a narrow pelvis, or if you have a large baby or twins.
• The diastasis may be larger if you are overweight or have poor abdominal tone.
• The abdominal hollowing exercise can help regain your figure.
• Vigorous abdominal training is dangerous after pregnancy.
• Correct posture is important after pregnancy to help prevent back pain.

Basic Concepts of Abdominal Training

Effective Muscle Strengthening

For a muscle to become stronger, it must be worked harder than it would be in everyday activities. When it is, we say that the muscle has been 'overloaded'. To achieve this degree of muscle work, we must decide on the type of exercise required, and its duration, frequency of use and intensity.

The type of exercise will dictate the type of strength we will build up. There are three major sorts of strength, termed 'isometric', 'concentric' and 'eccentric'. Isometric strength occurs when we tense a muscle and hold it tight. It is the type of strength needed to hold a joint still and to stop it moving. Concentric strength occurs when a muscle is shortening and speeding up a movement. It is the type used when we pick something up, for example. Eccentric strength is exactly the reverse. During eccentric activity the muscle begins to lengthen and is gradually 'let out'. It is the type of activity used when lowering a weight in a controlled fashion.

The three types of muscle work can be illustrated when standing up and sitting down in a chair. As we stand up the thigh muscles are tightening and working concentrically. If we stop ourselves just short of full standing and hold the position, the same muscles work isometrically. As we slowly lower ourselves down again back into the chair, the muscles are working eccentrically. All three types of muscle work are important to the abdominals, and so all three are used in the F.L.A.T. programme.

•••••••••••••••••• **KEYPOINT** ••••••••••••••••••
The three types of muscle action are concentric (lifting),
isometric (holding), and eccentric (lowering).

The intensity (how hard), duration (how long) and frequency (how often) of exercises used in the F.L.A.T. programme are also important. Too little exercise will fail to achieve the results we want. Too much will lead to overtraining, leaving us stale and possibly leading ultimately to injury. The intensity and duration of exercise are dictated by the type of muscles we are using. The abdominal muscles work mainly to tense and hold the trunk steady during everyday activities. To do this, the muscles will require endurance, so that they can continue to work for long periods. This may be achieved by working the muscles at slightly less than half of their maximum strength. When the muscles contract, we try to build up the length of time they can hold the contraction until eventually we can hold the abdominal muscles tight for 30 seconds or so.

Where the abdominal muscles are used in sport, in addition to their role of supporting the trunk by holding it tight, they may be used in dynamic actions to move the trunk rapidly. In this case, the muscles must be trained for power and speed. It is important to note that the supporting (stabilising) function of the abdominal muscles is always re-trained first in the F.L.A.T. programme. Only when this has been achieved, and an athlete has good control of trunk alignment and movement, should power movements begin. The restoration of good support in the trunk forms the foundation upon which other types of training may be built.

The frequency of practice will change as we progress through the programme. This is because initially the intention is to learn correct exercise technique. When learning technique, we aim for a high number of short practice bouts to help concentration. For the F.L.A.T. programme most exercises are practised twice daily to begin with. The only exception is abdominal hollowing which is practised regularly throughout the day during everyday activities. Once the techniques of the exercises have been mastered, the number of practice bouts reduces and the exercises become harder. Harder exercise will require a longer recovery period, and so exercises are now practised every other day, leaving a full day in-between to allow the muscles to recover.

• • • • • • • • • • • • • • • **KEYPOINT** • • • • • • • • • • • • • • • •
When deciding on an exercise, consider its type (which muscles are working), duration (how long it lasts), frequency (how often it is performed), and intensity (how hard it is).

THE PRINCIPLE OF TRAINING SPECIFICITY ● ● ● ● ● ● ● ● ● ●

When a muscle is strengthened, its make-up actually changes. The muscle becomes larger and tighter, and there are alterations in the chemicals it contains. In addition, the way the brain controls the movement itself becomes smoother and more co-ordinated. All of these changes constitute what we call the 'training adaptation'. In other words the changes which the body makes are a direct result of the training itself. The exact adaptation will closely reflect the type of exercise which has been used, and so we say that the muscle adaptation is 'specific' to the demands placed upon it.

An example from general sport may make this clearer. Imagine two people who run marathons. They want to reduce their times and go for a 'personal best'. If one person trains by running long distances and the other by running short sprints, who will be more successful in reducing their times? The answer is the person who runs distances. This type of training more accurately reflects the actions required during marathon running. Marathon runners need endurance. Short sprints will build mainly strength and speed, and so although the person using sprint training is getting fitter, the fitness is not the type required for the final marathon race. His body has changed (adapted) but these changes do not closely match those needed for running the marathon, they are not truly 'specific'.

● ● ● ● ● ● ● ● ● ● ● ● ● ● ● ● **KEYPOINT** ● ● ● ● ● ● ● ● ● ● ● ● ● ● ● ● ●
For an exercise to be truly 'specific' it must closely match the
action which we hope to improve.

When training the trunk muscles the same principles of specificity apply. We need to know what function the trunk muscles per-form, and then tailor our training programme to improve this function. We have already seen that trunk muscle function falls broadly into two categories, support or stabilisation, and move-ment. During stabilisation the trunk muscles work mainly isomet-rically (tense and hold) to make the trunk more solid. During movement the muscles work concentrically and eccentrically to perform actions such as bending and twisting. Importantly, however, the trunk must be stable before more rapid movements can be attempted, and our training should take this into account.

> •••••••••••••••• *KEYPOINT* ••••••••••••••••••
> The trunk muscles must be able to effectively hold the spine in
> a stable position before any vigorous trunk exercise is
> attempted.

During the F.L.A.T. programme we are aiming initially to restore the ability of the trunk muscles to stabilise the spine. Only when this has been achieved do we work on the muscles' ability to move the spine and provide power. For this reason, the initial part of the programme works the muscles responsible for stability and re-trains their ability to tense and hold the trunk still. At this stage, if rapid movements such as sit-ups are used, they could damage the spine. Rapid actions are not specific to stabilisation and until you are able to stabilise your spine and control it, rapid actions are dangerous.

Later, when stability has been re-trained, movements may begin. Initially they are slow and controlled and later they build up speed and power. At this later stage, the movements practised mimic the actions used in sport. In this way the training remains specific to a subject's individual sport.

> •••••••••••••••• *KEYPOINT* ••••••••••••••••••
> The F.L.A.T. programme begins by improving spinal stability
> and moves on to improve general movements.

FITNESS COMPONENTS •••••••••••••••••••••••••••••

Physical fitness may be defined as a person's ability to perform a physical task. Fitness may be seen on a continuum from an optimal level seen in the competitive athlete, through to the minimal standard required to stay healthy, and finally to a complete lack of fitness and the development of ill health (*see* fig. 15a). Fitness, then, is not simply a lack of disease, it is more than this. It is the ability of the body to allow a person to live a happy and well balanced life.

We can think of fitness in two parts. There is health-related fitness which involves items directly related to improving health and preventing disease. But also, there is task- or performance-related fitness which involves factors necessary for a person to perform a particular sport, or an activity at work for example. To make things easier we can divide fitness into a series of components or 'S' factors (*see* fig. 15b).

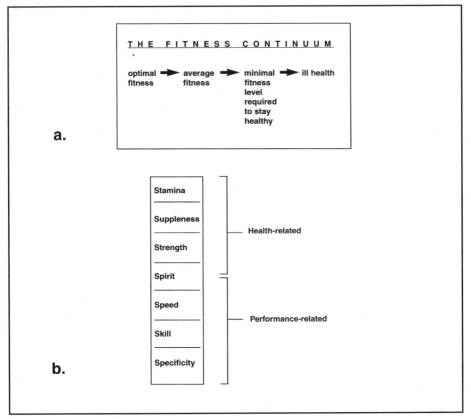

Fig. 15 *Physical fitness*

• **Stamina** encompasses heart–lung fitness and also muscle endurance, or the ability to keep an exercise going.
• **Suppleness** (flexibility) and **Strength** are both essential to the health of the joints.
• **Spirit** involves psychological factors which are important to both health and sport, such as motivation, how satisfied a person is with their own body, and a positive outlook on life.
• **Speed** (also encompassing power) is needed for explosive actions in sport.
• **Skill** is important to all actions, but especially those involving complex movements.
• **Specificity**, as we have seen, is important when matching exercise to sports actions.

The important point about the components of fitness is that they must be balanced. Often, exercise works on one component but not on others. For example, intensive bodybuilding may provide dramatic gains in strength, but little improvement in suppleness or stamina. Running marathons will generate a high degree of stamina, but little suppleness or strength in the upper body.

When the fitness components become imbalanced, the body may be pulled out of alignment and injury can result. For example, if muscles are strong but not supple they will tend to pull or 'strain' more easily. If a joint is too supple it will have little stability and may give way. The aim with fitness is to improve all components more or less equally.

> •••••••••••••••• **KEYPOINT** ••••••••••••••••••
> All the fitness components must be balanced for optimal health.

Skill is often a fitness component which is forgotten. In the race to lift heavier weights, to stretch further or run faster, the quality of an exercise frequently takes a back seat to quantity. But as with so many things in life, more is not necessarily better. If the quality of a movement suffers, injury is more likely because an action becomes clumsy. In the F.L.A.T. programme we are aiming for *quality* of movement before quantity with every single exercise. The initial movements aim to re-educate the basic skills of spinal movement which have often lain dormant since childhood. This is essential because it forms the foundation for the whole programme. A person must be able to perform an exercise in a smooth, controlled fashion before the number of repetitions is increased.

> ••••••••••••••• **KEYPOINT** ••••••••••••••••••
> The quality (control) of an exercise is more important than the
> quantity (number of repetitions) that can be performed.

CONTROLLING THE NEUTRAL SPINAL POSITION • • • • • • • •

One of the most basic movements that you will need to control is pelvic tilting. You must be able to recognise when the pelvis tilts and pulls the spine out of alignment during everyday activities. As we have seen, the ideal alignment of the spine is a position where the pelvis is mid-way between being tilted fully back and fully forwards (*see* page 10). We call this the 'neutral position'. In the neutral position, the joints, discs, and tissues are subjected to loads which they were designed to withstand. When we move away from the neutral position, stress on some tissues reduces but stress on others increases dramatically. The neutral position is therefore a 'safety zone' for the spine.

The practical methods used to find the neutral position covered elsewhere (*see* pages 10 and 42). Once you have mastered the neutral position, use it regularly throughout the day and during all exercises. Try to sit in a chair with your spine in its neutral position. If you are in a gym using weight training apparatus, perform the exercise with your spine in its neutral position. When you are using stretching exercises, again try to keep the spine in its neutral position for as long as possible.

• • • • • • • • • • • • • • • **KEYPOINT** • • • • • • • • • • • • • • • •
The spine is in its neutral position when the pelvis is level and the lower back is slightly hollow. Use the neutral position as often as possible to safeguard your back.

PROGRESSIVE EXERCISE ●

We have seen that to train the body we must overload it; that is, make the body work harder than it would normally during everyday activities. However, as fitness improves, the same amount of activity becomes easier and no longer taxes the body to the same degree. The training effect therefore reduces. To maintain the overload and continue to work the body sufficiently, the exercise must get harder as we become fitter. We now say that the exercise is 'progressing'.

• • • • • • • • • • • • • • • **KEYPOINT** • • • • • • • • • • • • • • • •
Over time, as an exercise becomes easier we must progress it (make it harder) to maintain the training effect.

One of the ways of progressing a weight training exercise is to perform a greater number of lifts (repetitions) with each training session. To progress stamina when running, we could simply run a longer distance with each training session. But there are other methods of progressing an exercise without increasing the amount of training that we do.

One such method of progressing an exercise is to increase the degree of leverage the body is subjected to. In a sit-up action, for example, if the arms are held by the sides the weight of the upper body acts in the centre of the trunk, and the distance between the pivot point of the action (the hip joint) and the weight of the body represents a lever. If the arms are placed behind the head, their weight has moved away from the pivot point and so the leverage effect is greater. If the arms are held above the head, again the leverage has increased so the exercise has progressed (*see* fig. 16). In each case the weight of the body has obviously remained the same, but the increasing leverage effect has placed an additional overload on the working muscles.

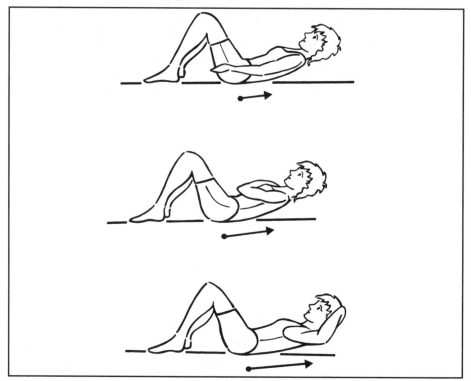

Fig. 16 *Progressing an exercise using leverage. As the arms move higher up the body, the leverage distance between the hip and arm weight increases*

A second method of exercise progression is to change the type of work a muscle has to perform. When a muscle is working against a load, for example when trying to lift a weight, it can work in three ways. If the muscle can create enough force to move the load, it is working concentrically. If it can only create enough force to hold the load still it is working isometrically. If it can't lift the weight or even hold it, but can make the weight lower more slowly, it is working eccentrically. An eccentric action is therefore easier than an isometric action and this in turn is easier than a concentric action. If a muscle is very weak we should therefore begin with eccentric or isometric work (lowering or holding) before we move on to concentric work (lifting).

Adding resistance is another method of exercise progression for strength. The resistance may be anything which makes the movement harder. Elastic bands, springs, weights, and even the resistance of moving through water, will all strengthen muscle more effectively than free movement.

TARGETING THE DEEP MUSCLE CORSET • • • • • • • • • • •

To improve core stability we need to use the deep corset muscles local to the spine – transversus, internal obliques and multifidus – and the more general muscles which we have termed as 'global'. The F.L.A.T. programme focuses on the local muscles first, and only when they are functioning normally do we begin to work the more general global muscles – in particular, the back and side back muscles (spinal extensors and quadratus lumborum), buttocks (gluteals), thigh muscles (quadriceps) and the powerful shoulder 'pulling' muscles (trapezius and rhomboids which retract the shoulder and latissimus dorsi). In each case, when working these powerful global muscles, alignment will be maintained by using the new-found core stability.

One of the reasons we focus on the deep muscle corset first is that these muscles may actually have forgotten how to work! If a person has suffered from back pain, or if they have had surgery where the tummy has been cut, the muscles may not work correctly. After pregnancy the muscles may take time to 'switch back on', and if a person is very overweight or very inactive the muscles may not have been used for a long time. In each of these cases the deep muscle corset may not be functioning correctly and so we have to 'wake up' or 'switch on' the muscles before we can continue to train them with exercise.

•••••••••••••••••• *KEYPOINT* ••••••••••••••••••
The F.LA.T. programme focuses on getting the deep corset
muscles working again, before other forms of exercise
are used.

The transversus and internal oblique muscles pull the abdomen in. They do not bend the trunk as with a sit-up action. The sit-up action works the rectus muscle in the centre of the abdomen and the external obliques at the side. When these two powerful muscles work, they tend to dominate the movement and eclipse the action of the deep corset. To be able to restore the deep corset, therefore, the exercises must work these muscles in isolation. The action involves gently pulling the tummy button in, without bending the spine or moving the rib cage. For good core stability these muscles must also be able to hold themselves tight for a long period. Rather than building the exercise up and making it harder with weights or bands (resistance), for example, you gradually increase the time that the muscles can hold themselves tight (endurance). In a gym, an athlete may build up the arm muscles by gradually increasing the weight that is lifted, starting, for example, with 10 kg and moving up to 15 kg or 20 kg. This type of training is not suitable for the deep muscle corset. Instead, you tighten the muscles and initially hold them tight for 1 second, before gradually building up this holding time to 5 seconds or 10 seconds, all the time breathing normally and certainly not holding the breath.

••••••••••••••• *KEYPOINT* ••••••••••••••••••
To target the corset muscles rather than the 'sit-up' muscles,
gently pull the tummy button in and hold the contraction, without bending the spine or moving the rib cage.

Posture

Posture is simply the relationship or 'alignment' between the various parts of the body. It is important from two standpoints. Firstly, good posture underlies all exercise techniques. Your posture is really your foundation for movement. In the same way that a building will fall down if its foundations are shaky, your whole body will suffer if your posture is poor. Exercises which begin from the basis of poor posture tend to be awkward and clumsy. Because of this they are less effective and, more importantly, the person using awkward, clumsy movements is likely to be injured.

The second important point about posture is that an incorrect posture allows physical stress to build up in certain tissues, ultimately leading to pain and injury. For example, a person who is very round-shouldered may simply have started out with tightness in the chest muscles and weakness in the muscles which brace the shoulders back. If this combination had been corrected at the time, the poor posture may not have built up over the years. As a consequence of poor posture, the way that the joints move will change. Alteration in movement of this type will mean that joints can be subjected to uneven stresses. When this continues over the years, the eventual outcome can be the development of 'osteoarthritis' in later life.

We saw earlier that fitness is really a combination of various components which we called 'S' factors. In relation to posture the two most important fitness components are flexibility and strength. Postural changes are often associated with poor muscle tone (weakness) in some muscles together with too much tone (tightening) in others. This imbalance in tone gives an uneven pull from the muscles around a joint, and causes the joint to move off-centre (see fig. 17). Our aim with exercise is to redress the balance in muscle tone by using stretching exercises to lengthen tight muscles, combined with strengthening exercises to increase the tone of lax muscles.

● ● ● ● ● ● ● ● ● ● ● ● ● ● *KEYPOINT* ● ● ● ● ● ● ● ● ● ● ● ● ● ●
Your posture will affect the way you exercise, and the
exercises you choose will in turn alter your posture.

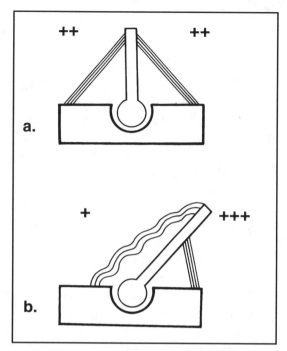

Fig. 17 *Posture and muscle imbalance: (a) normal joint – equal muscle tone gives correct joint alignment; (b) postural imbalance – unequal muscle tone pulls joint out of alignment*

OPTIMAL POSTURE

We cannot talk about a normal posture because very few people are 'normal' in the true sense of the word. Equally, if we talk about an average posture, the average may be very poor and this type of posture is far from ideal. Instead we should talk about an 'optimal' posture, where the various body segments are aligned correctly, and the minimum of stress is placed on the body tissues. This type of posture requires little muscle activity to maintain it because it is essentially balanced.

The various segments of the body work together like the links in a chain. Movement in one causes movement in the next link which is then passed on to the next, and so on. This means that a postural change in one part of the body can alter the alignment of another body part quite far away. Alterations in the feet are a good illustration of this point. Flat feet, where the inner arch of the foot moves downwards, will in turn twist the shinbone and then the thighbone. Eventually these changes can be felt in the lower back, chest and neck. Because of this intimate link between body segments, it is important to correct any postural fault, however minor it may seem at the time.

•••••••••••••••• ***KEYPOINT*** ••••••••••••••••
In an optimal posture the body segments are correctly aligned, so very little effort is needed to maintain the position.

One method of looking at posture is to compare it to the posture line. In an optimal posture this line is similar to a plumb line dropped vertically downwards from the top of the head. The body should be evenly distributed along this line (*see* fig. 18), and ideally the line should pass just in front of the knee, travel through the hip and shoulder joints and through the ear. Looking more closely at the pelvis, optimal pelvic alignment occurs when the lip of the pelvis is in a direct vertical line with the pubic bone in the groin. In this position there should be a gentle curve to the lumbar spine and a gentle curve to the neck. However, various alterations occur from this normal posture line with which we need to concern ourselves.

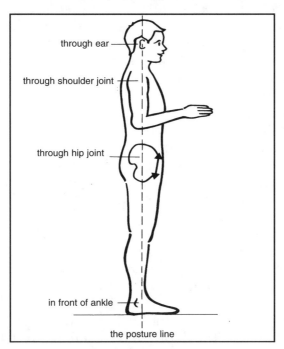

through ear

through shoulder joint

through hip joint

in front of ankle

the posture line

Fig. 18 *Optimal posture: the lip of the pelvis forms a near-vertical line with the pubic bone in the groin*

ASSESSING YOUR OWN POSTURE ● ● ● ● ● ● ● ● ● ● ● ● ● ● ●

Before you can correct posture using the F.L.A.T. exercises, you must determine your current body alignment. You will need to work with a partner; they will assess your posture and you in turn will assess theirs. Ask your partner to stand against a straight vertical edge, such as a doorframe, or plumb line attached to a hook. Make sure that the edge of the line is slightly in front of their anklebone and then compare their posture to this reference line. Fig. 18 shows the posture line, together with the optimal alignment. Photocopy this diagram, and then mark on the sheet the positions of their knee, hip, shoulder and ear. It is the centre point of each of these that we are interested in. The next step is to determine the position of your partner's pelvis. Draw an imaginary line from the rim of the pelvis (the furthest point forwards) to their pubic bone. Determine whether this line is vertical or positioned at an angle.

Once you have assessed your partner's posture from the side, turn them around so that their back is towards you. Their feet should be about 10 cm (4 in.) apart. We will now continue the postural assessment using fig. 19. Start by looking at the feet. The inner edge of the foot should have a gentle arch, and should not be flat. Moving up the leg, the Achilles tendon should be vertical and the bulk of the calf muscles should be equal. The creases on the back of the knees and the lower edge of the buttocks should be on the same level for both sides of the body. The pelvis itself should be level horizontally and the spine aligned vertically. One of the ways that spinal alignment can be checked is to look at the skin creases on either side of the lower trunk; they should be equal in number and shape. The shoulder blades should be about three finger-breadths (6–8 cm) apart, and they should lie on the same horizontal line. The contours of the shoulders should be on the same level and they should appear similar in size and shape. Finally, the head should be level and not tilted to one side. Record any changes from the optimal posture on a photocopy of fig. 19.

The final method of posture assessment is to establish the depth of the curve in the lower back. Ideally, the curve should be gently hollow. When it is too deep, or too flat, the alignment of the lumbar region changes, indicating that the pelvic tilt is no longer correct. Assess the depth of the lumbar curve by standing with your back up against a wall. Stand with the feet 15–20 cm (6–8 in.) from the wall and the buttocks and shoulders touching

	POSITION OF BODY PART	YOUR SCORE
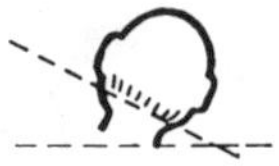	Head position	
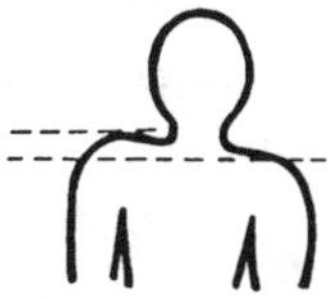	Shoulder level	
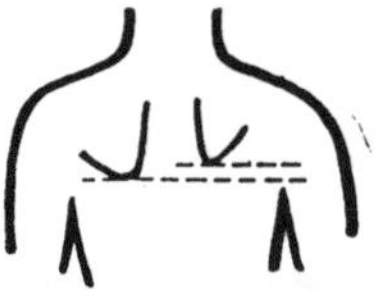	Position of shoulder blade contour	
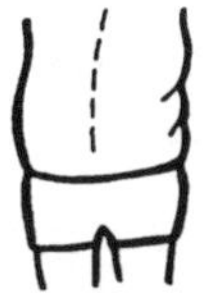	Skin creases at waist and spinal alignment	
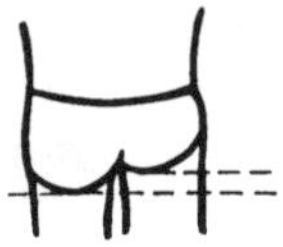	Level of buttock creases	
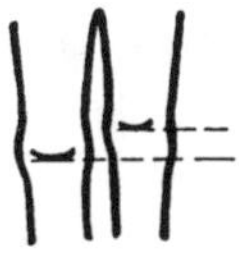	Level of knee creases	
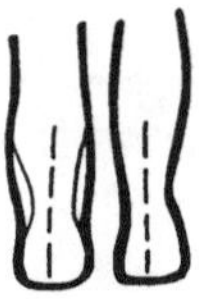	Calf muscle bulk and Achilles alignment	
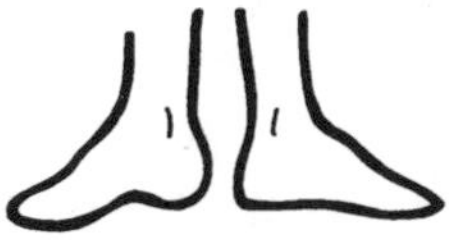	Flat foot or high arch	

Fig. 19 *Assessing standing posture from behind*

the wall (*see* fig. 20). Have your partner slide their hand between the wall and the small of your back. Ideally they should be able to push the hand through the gap only as far as the fingers (*see* fig. 20a). If the whole hand passes through (*see* fig. 20b), your lumbar curve is too deep. If they can only get the tips of the fingers between your back and the wall, the lumbar curve is too flat (*see* fig. 20c).

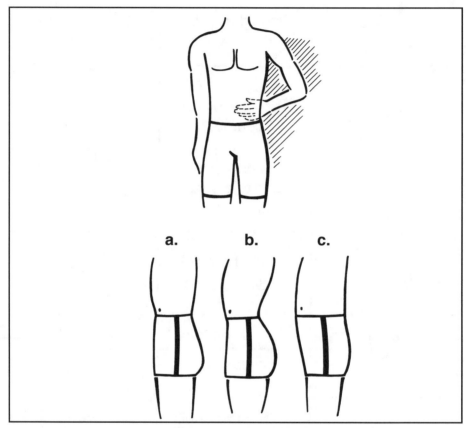

Fig. 20 *Assessing the lumbar curve: (a) normal; (b) too deep; (c) too flat*

SUMMARY

In an optimal posture:
- the hip, shoulder and ear lie in a vertical line
- the pelvis is level
- the lower spine should be gently hollowed
- the inner edge of the shoulder blades are 6–8 cm (3 in.) apart.

HOLLOW BACK POSTURE •

In an optimal posture the pelvis should be level, with the front rim of the pelvis and the pubic bone in a vertical line when viewed from the side. In this position the lower part of the back (the lumbar spine) should be slightly hollowed. In the hollow back posture, however, the abdominal muscles become weak and lengthened, allowing the pelvis to tip forwards. When this happens the pull on the lumbar spine increases the lumbar curve. This increased curvature places stress on the discs and small joints (facet joints) of the lower spine. Over time, back pain can result. This can be particularly bad if a person stands for long periods.

The problem here is not abdominal strength but the length of the abdominal muscles, and the fact that the lower spine has been held in its hollow position for a long time. To correct the hollow back posture we must choose exercises which aim to shorten the abdominals. The abdominal hollowing exercises and trunk curl are the two which we use in the programme, and are described on pages 86–9 and 98 respectively. This type of posture is particularly common after pregnancy and is also seen in young female gymnasts, who choose this posture to walk.

The hollow back posture (*see* fig. 21a) is the classic 'beer belly' posture where many years of inactivity, combined with excess weight, leave the abdominals poorly toned. Often the angulation of the pelvis can shorten the hip flexor muscles and these will require stretching. The exercise for this is shown in fig. 21b. Initially the person takes up a half-kneeling position and they perform the abdominal hollowing exercise to tighten and stabilise their trunk. From this position they then press themselves forwards, forcing their lower leg into extension, effectively stretching the hip flexors. It is essential when this exercise is performed that the lower spine does not hollow. When this happens the movement is occurring at the lumbar spine rather than the hip.

Where the posture has been present for many years, the base of the spine may be very stiff. Fig. 21c shows an exercise to relieve this stiffness. Lie flat on the floor with your knees bent. Grip your legs behind your knees and pull the knees up towards the chest. This will have the effect of rounding the lower spine in the opposite direction to the hollow back. Make sure that the movement is slow and controlled. Never force the spine to move if it is stiff, but encourage it gently.

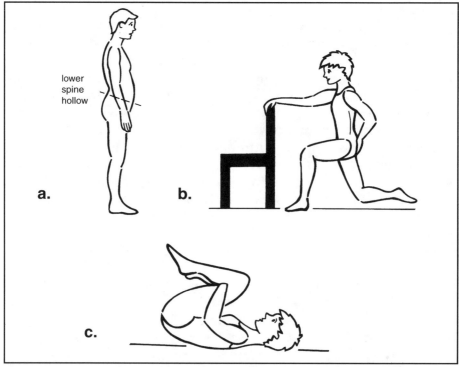

Fig. 21 *Hollow back posture: (a) abdominal muscles sag; (b) hip flexor stretch; (c) knee-to-chest back stretch*

•••••••••••••••• **KEYPOINT** ••••••••••••••••
In the hollow back posture, the lumbar curve is excessive and the abdominal muscles are lengthened.

HEAD, NECK AND SHOULDER POSTURE ● ● ● ● ● ● ● ● ● ● ● ●

Head and neck posture are important considerations when using abdominal exercises. Often standard sit-up movements, placing the hands behind the neck, can lead to the development of poor posture in this region and subsequent pain.

When we look at a person from the side, their shoulder joint and ear should be positioned on the posture line. A common postural abnormality associated with the upper spine is called the round back posture (*see* fig. 22). Changes occur in the position of the head and neck, the shoulder joint and upper (thoracic) spine. The normal curve of the thoracic region is lost and pain often develops between the shoulder blades.

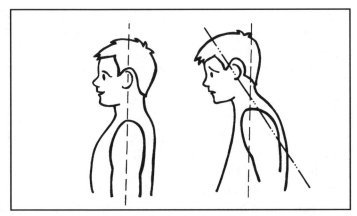

Fig. 22 *Round back posture: normal (left); incorrect head and shoulder alignment (right)*

When we look at a person from the side, if they have the round back posture the head is often held forwards with the shoulders being excessively rounded. The chest muscles ('pectorals') are normally too tight, while the muscles that pull the shoulders back ('retractors') are often too weak. Looking at the person from the back, the shoulder blades should be roughly 6–8 cm (3 in.) apart. However, in the round back posture, weakness of the shoulder muscles allows the shoulder blades to drop apart and to twist.

These posture exercises aim to stretch the tight chest muscles, strengthen the weak shoulder muscles, and stretch the muscles at the back of the neck. The first exercise we use to achieve this is shown in fig. 23. A person lies flat on the floor with their arms

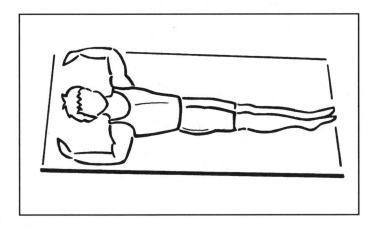

Fig. 23 *Chest stretch*

spread into a 'T' shape. From this position the elbows are bent and the arms take up a 90° position. Simply holding this position will stretch the chest muscles and the muscles which twist the shoulders. Breathe slowly and try to relax into the movement.

To strengthen the upper back muscles a similar position is taken up, but this time lying on the front. Again the person stretches their arms out into a 'T' shape but this time they stay straight. The aim now is simply to lift the straight arms up by 5 cm (2 in.) and to hold that position for 10 seconds (*see* fig. 24). This will bring the shoulder blades together and strengthen the muscles surrounding these areas. Perform this movement five times, each time holding the position for 10 seconds.

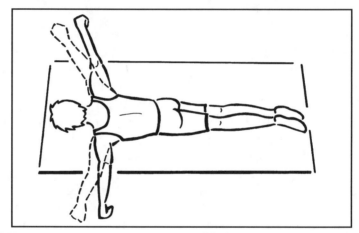

Fig. 24 *Strengthening the 'retractor' muscles in the upper back*

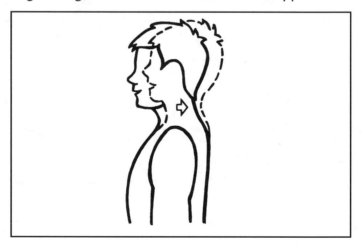

Fig. 25 *Drawing the head backwards, tucking the chin in*

To stretch the neck muscles, perform a chin tuck movement. Stand upright with the head level. From this position, simply draw the chin inwards without looking up or down (*see* fig. 25). This allows the neck to move on a single line, allowing the joints in the neck to glide freely. As you pull the chin in, the curve at the base of the neck is flattened and you should feel the muscles behind the neck stretching.

• • • • • • • • • • • • • • • • *KEYPOINT* • • • • • • • • • • • • • • • • •
In the round back posture the chin pokes forwards, and the shoulders are rounded. The chest muscles are tight, and the muscles controlling the shoulder blades are weak.

SWAYBACK POSTURE •

We have seen that to assess posture we compare a person's body alignment to a vertical plumb line. In the swayback posture, the pelvis stays level but the hips move forwards of the posture line (*see* fig. 26). Because the hip joint now lies in front of the posture line, the hip is effectively pulled back into extension. In this position the hip flexor muscles are lengthened, exactly the opposite situation to that which we saw in the hollow back posture earlier (*see* page 43).

If we compare the normal and swayback postures, we can see that in a normal posture the furthest point forwards is the chest, while the furthest point backwards are the buttocks. In the swayback, however, the furthest point forwards is the abdomen, and the thoracic spine is the furthest point back. Looking at the lower back in the normal posture, the lumbar curve is gently hollow along its whole length. In the swayback, however, the hollow is sharp and more pronounced in the lower region of the spine. Finally, in the normal posture the spine and leg are close to the posture line, but in the swayback the spine and leg form a curve with the person's whole body profile taking on the shape of a letter 'V' turned on its side. The swayback is a relaxed or slumped posture frequently seen in adolescents.

Correction of the swayback posture is accomplished through continuous practice of correct alignment rather than strength or stretching exercises. Because the bodyline in the swayback is curved, a person with this posture appears shorter. Simply by trying to stand tall, the swayback should correct itself.

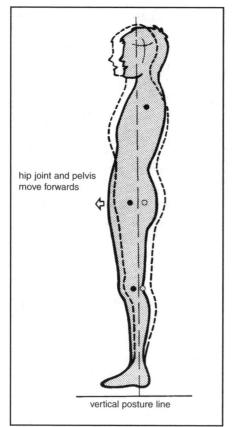

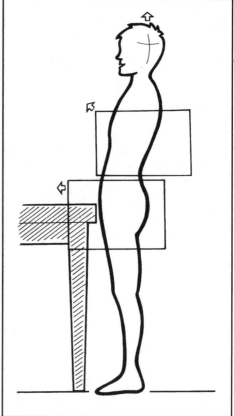

Fig. 26 *Swayback posture*

Fig. 27 *Correction of swayback posture. Stand in front of a table. The chest moves forward and the spine is lengthened. Stand 'tall'*

Further improvement is achieved by practising correct body segment alignment with particular reference to the pelvis. Stand in front of a table with the edge of the table just touching the pelvis. Imagine your pelvis and chest to be two separate blocks (*see* fig. 27). Without bending, slide your chest forwards, trying to avoid pressing your pelvis harder into the table.

• • • • • • • • • • • • • • • **KEYPOINT** • • • • • • • • • • • • • • • •
In the swayback posture the hip and pelvis are thrust forwards, and the body slouches.

FLATBACK POSTURE •

In the flatback posture, a person shows a markedly reduced lumbar curve. When standing straight with the spine up against a wall, you should normally be able to place the flat of your hand between the wall and your lower spine (see fig. 20, page 42). Someone with a flatback posture may only be able to place one or two fingers in the gap formed. In this posture, the pelvis has tilted backwards and the lumbar spine has been pulled with it. The flatback is commonly seen where a person has spent a lot of time sitting slumped in a chair. It is particularly common after a bout of back pain where a person has rested in bed for too long. Stiffness may occur either when bending forwards or bending backwards, with the spine becoming almost fixed in the flatback position.

Stretching can help to alleviate the pain from this condition, providing it is performed gently to encourage movement rather than to force it. The stretching should feel slightly uncomfortable because the exercises are working on very tight structures. However, they should not give back pain, and in cases where this occurs exercise should only be carried out under the supervision of a physiotherapist. Start the stretch by lying flat on your front. Place your forearms down on the floor at the side of your chest. Keeping your hips down, push with your arms and arch the spine until you come up on your forearms (*see* fig. 28). Practise the exercise each day, and gradually the movement will come back.

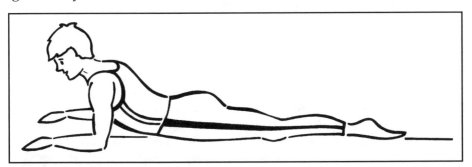

Fig. 28 *Correction of flatback posture*

• • • • • • • • • • • • • • • • *KEYPOINT* • • • • • • • • • • • • • • • • •
In the flatback posture the normal lumbar curve is lost, and the lower back appears stiff.

Diet and Exercise

People often begin using abdominal exercises in the hope of reducing their waistline. They join a local gym or exercise class and work hard for many months. Eventually, however, they can lose enthusiasm if they fail to see the results they wanted. Instead of reducing their waistline all they have achieved is a marginal re-shaping, and they give up exercising, disillusioned. There are two reasons for the failure of this type of training. Firstly, if exercise is not coupled with a correct diet, you will not lose significant amounts of weight. Secondly, the type of training will determine the effect it has on your waistline. The wrong type of training will often have little effect at all.

Bodyweight and body fat

People often talk about being overweight, meaning that they have too much loose flesh around the abdomen (men), and around the abdomen, thighs and buttocks (women). However, your bodyweight is made up of a number of things. Bone, muscle, fluids, body organs, fat and other tissues all contribute to your total weight. Take a sauna and you will lose weight because you sweat out water, but this is not a permanent weight loss. Begin a weight training programme and your muscles will become sleek, firm and toned. This may be desirable, but because muscle weighs more than fat you may actually gain a few pounds. What we really mean when we say someone is overweight is that they have too much fat, possibly linked to flabby muscle.

Body fat occurs in different types. Essential body fat is found around the body organs and within the marrow in the centre of the bones. Women have more fat than men because they carry additional sex-specific fat which is important for a variety of hormonal functions. If the level of fat is reduced too much, as can be the case in young girls who diet excessively, for example, a woman's periods will often stop due to the hormonal changes caused by the low body fat. The other type of fat is storage fat which is found beneath the skin and acts as a depot for energy. It is the storage fat which often becomes excessive.

In order to lose inches from the waistline we need to reduce the amount of body fat, while maintaining a healthy, balanced diet. But this must be coupled with exercise to tone and shape the muscles of the abdomen or they will remain flabby.

•••••••••••••••• *KEYPOINT* ••••••••••••••••••
The amount of body fat you have is more important than your weight.

THE FEEDING CONTROL MECHANISM ● ● ● ● ● ● ● ● ● ● ● ● ●

One of the main factors which assists in the control of an ideal bodyweight is the 'feeding control mechanism' (F.C.M.). This is situated within the brain in an area called the 'hypothalamus'. The F.C.M. controls bodyweight by matching the amount of energy obtained from food to the requirements of the body through activity. If the amount of energy going into the body is exactly equal to the amount going out, the bodyweight will remain constant. Individuals who are overweight tend to have lost the ability to precisely match their energy requirements to their diet. Unless the F.C.M. is re-set, long-term control of an ideal bodyweight is unlikely. One of the problems with crash diets is that although they lead to a short-term reduction in weight, because they restrict the amount of energy going in, the F.C.M. tries to conserve energy and the 'tick-over speed' of the body (the 'basal metabolic rate') is slowed by as much as 45%. This means that weight loss will slow down and a person can quickly lose motivation because they always desire more food than they are getting. When they stop the diet the weight goes back on again and we get a yo-yo effect of repeated weight loss and weight gain over a period of time.

A more effective method of weight control is to combine good dietary habits with regular activity, as this type of programme has been shown to re-set the F.C.M. to the correct levels.

A NOTE ON CALORIES ●

The energy taken into the body as food, and that expended during activity, is measured in calories, a measure of the heat a food would produce if it were burnt. One kilocalorie or Calorie (with a capital 'C') is the more common measure, and this is equivalent to 4.2 joules, the joule being the other measure of food energy seen on food packaging. Some of the main constituents of food are carbohydrate, a starchy or sugary material giving energy, fat, an energy store, and protein, used to build the body tissues. All of these substances can be used by the body for energy, and so may be measured in Calories. Both carbohydrate and protein produce the same amount of energy. Fat is a more concentrated energy source, and can produce more than double the energy of the other two foods. This is why fat is used as an energy store, and reducing it from the diet is a good way to lose weight. Another source of energy is alcohol which has almost the same number of Calories as fat.

Foods are made up of a mixture of nutrients, and so we give each food a total Calorie value, reflecting the proportional amounts of the various nutrients it contains. The Calorie value is useful when the food is used as part of a Calorie-controlled diet to lose weight, but does not relate to the quality of the food. This is because high-Calorie foods are not necessarily high in vitamins and minerals, and fibre contains virtually no Calories at all, but is still an important part of the diet.

Energy is used up by the body in two ways. Even without movement, the body has a certain 'resting energy' requirement for breathing, heartbeat, digestion and other bodily functions. The amount of energy needed for these processes can vary from person to person depending on many factors, including body size. This resting energy is the basal metabolic rate, and normally uses up about 1200 Calories each day. The other requirement for energy comes from 'voluntary activity', including things such as manual work and exercise. People who have active jobs, and those who exercise intensely, will burn up more Calories.

Different sports will burn off Calories at different rates. For example, slow jogging may use 120 Calories an hour, while driving a car needs only 48 Calories. Intense swimming or circuit weight training, where all the muscles are worked, can use over 250 Calories in the same time. In order to significantly burn Calories, the exercise should be continuous for 20–30 minutes and must be practised regularly.

LOSING WEIGHT ●

When the amount of energy taken into the body from food equals the amount being expended during exercise and everyday activities, we can say that a person is in 'energy balance'. In this situation they will neither gain nor lose weight. If the energy input is greater than the expenditure, the extra energy will be stored as fat. If too little energy is taken in, the body makes up the deficit by drawing on stored energy and burning up fat.

•••••••••••••••• *KEYPOINT* ••••••••••••••••
When the amount of energy coming into your body as food
equals the amount going out through activity and exercise, you
are said to be in 'energy balance'.

Clearly, one of the methods of losing weight is simply to eat
less. However, this has a number of disadvantages for those
exercising regularly. Firstly, it is more difficult to eat a
sufficient quantity of nutrients; secondly, tissue other than fat
is lost, particularly with extreme weight loss diets. At the onset
of a diet, 70% of weight loss is from water (*see* fig. 29), reducing
to about 20% by the time a person has been dieting for two
weeks. Fat loss speeds up as the diet is continued, changing
from 25% of the total weight loss in the early days of a diet, to
about 70% after two weeks. Protein loss increases from 5% to
15% in the same timescale.

Rather than crash dieting then, a better method is to improve
the general quality of the diet. It is not just the amount of food,
but the type of food which is important. High-energy foods
(those with a lot of Calories, especially fat and alcohol) should
be restricted, and these should be replaced with low-Calorie
equivalents. The total amount of food may remain the same. It is
important not to reduce the carbohydrate foods too much as
these provide both the energy for exercise, and necessary
amounts of fibre. It is more important to reduce the high-fat
foods, and use a low-fat/high-carbohydrate diet.

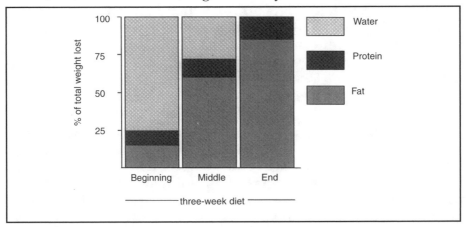

Fig. 29 *Relative contributions of water, protein and fat to total weight
lost during a three-week diet*

The essential items to restrict are alcohol, fast foods such as French fries and crisps, and snacks such as chocolate, because these are high in fat. Trim all visible fat and grill rather than fry food. Use less refined foods such as wholemeal bread and cereals, and eat starchy foods such as potatoes and pasta rather than sweet foods for energy.

CAN EXERCISE HELP YOU LOSE WEIGHT?

There are a number of myths about exercise and weight loss which we need to dispel. It is often said that if you start exercising your appetite will increase and you will put on weight. This is not so. Regular exercise helps to re-set the feeding control mechanism. Studies have shown that those who exercise regularly have a greater ability to accurately match the amount of food they want with the amount their body actually needs. This is especially important in children. Scientific studies have consistently shown that inactive children are more likely to be overweight in later life.

A second myth concerns the ability of exercise to burn off fat. You will hear people say that you would have to exercise all day to burn off the pounds they need to lose. After all, to lose just 0.45 kg (1 lb) of bodyweight you would have to chop wood for 10 hours or play volleyball for 32 hours! However, this type of argument fails to take into account the regularity of exercise. Although only a small number of Calories are burned with each exercise bout, the cumulative effect is great. If, for example, you were to play two hours of golf, it would take four to five weeks to burn off 0.45 kg of fat. But, if you play each week for the whole year, you will have burnt off over 6 kg (nearly a stone) in total – a very significant amount!

Coupling exercise with a good diet is the best route to permanent weight loss. As mentioned, exercise helps to re-set the F.C.M., and the desire to eat too much is reduced. Secondly, exercise speeds up the metabolic rate – the 'ticking over' of the body – so that even when exercise has finished, energy will continue to be burned off. A half-hour workout, for example, will continue to burn up Calories for three or four hours afterwards. Of course, exercise will not just reduce weight but will increase muscle tone and add greatly to the overall improvement in physical appearance.

```
•••••••••••••••• KEYPOINT •••••••••••••••••
Regular exercise is essential to effective, long-term weight loss.
```

BODY TYPE

People often compare themselves to others to determine if they are satisfied with their body. Are they too big or too small, too fat or too thin? Is their waistline OK? Are their hips too big? Although this is understandable, one of the problems is that we each have a different body type. In other words, your body is unique, and the only way to judge if you are in good shape is to know what feels and looks good for you.

The shape of the human body can be classified into three distinct types (*see* fig. 30). The first type is angular ('mesomorph'). This type of body tends to be muscular, with a typical 'Tarzan' appearance: the shoulders are broad and the waist is slim. These people tend to have large bones and thick-set muscles. The second type is more rounded ('endomorph') and represented by the 'Billy Bunter' shape. These individuals have a smooth, soft outline with a 'peardrop' appearance. The waist and chest are often roughly the same measurement, and fat is carried on the upper arms and thighs as well as around the waist. The third type is linear ('ectomorph') represented by the typical 'bean poles'. These individuals tend to be tall and thin, with long legs and arms. Their muscles are long and fine, and they have a wiry appearance.

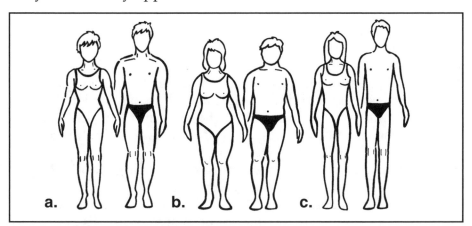

Fig. 30 *Body types: (a) mesomorph – muscular; (b) endomorph – rounded; (c) ectomorph – linear*

55

In reality, we are all a mixture of these three extremes. But the proportion of each body type you have will determine your overall shape, and there is little you can do to change this.

Take as an example a young girl with a very rounded, stout appearance. She sees models in the fashion magazines who are tall and thin with long delicate limbs. Wanting to change her appearance she joins a local aerobics class and starts dieting. Initially her weight reduces but she becomes unhappy because she feels she is not achieving what she wanted. She is fitter, and her muscles are more toned, but she does not look like the magazine models. Why? Not because she has failed to work hard enough, but because she has a different body type. She has a mixture of the rounded (endomorph) and angular (mesomorph) physiques, while the magazine model has a linear (ectomorph) body type. This young girl is now fit and toned. She should be happy, energetic and carefree. Instead she is depressed and self-conscious because she is aiming to change the body type she was born with. This is impossible. It is far better to achieve the best you can for your own body than to want someone else's!

• • • • • • • • • • • • • • • • **KEYPOINT** • • • • • • • • • • • • • • • • •
Our bodies combine tendencies towards being fat, lean and muscled. The combination of these factors you were born with determines your body type.

For further information on diet and exercise *see* Anita Bean's *The Complete Guide to Sports Nutrition.*

SUMMARY

• Body fat is a more important consideration than bodyweight. This includes muscle, bone, tissues and fluids as well as fat.
• The feeding control mechanism (F.C.M.) in the brain attempts to match the amount of energy you take in as food to the amount you burn off through physical activity.
• Starches and sugars are energy-providing foods called carbohydrates. Fat is an energy store and is high in Calories.
• Your basal metabolic rate (B.M.R.) is the 'tick-over rate' of your body. Exercise increases this, re-activates your F.C.M., and increases muscle tone.
• You cannot change the body type you were born with.

COMMON ABDOMINAL EXERCISES

One of the aims of the F.L.A.T. programme is to improve the standard of abdominal exercises, and in so doing to make exercises for this body part both safer and more effective. To fulfil this aim, the first thing we need to do is to take a close look at some commonly practised exercises and see where these go wrong. Although many of these have been practised for many years in numerous gyms and exercise classes, there is still much room for improvement.

THE SIT-UP

The sit-up is often the first exercise turned to when abdominal training is considered. Unfortunately this exercise has a number of inherent dangers, especially for the spine. By knowing what happens to the body during this action we can reduce these dangers considerably.

Begin the exercise lying flat on your back. As soon as you lift your head from the floor, the abdominal muscles begin to work. This is because the muscles lifting the neck pull on the rib cage. To stop the ribs from moving, and hold them firm, the abdominal muscles must tighten. As the exercise continues, you begin to lift your trunk from the floor. To do this, your legs have to stay down. However, because your legs are lighter than your trunk, the tendency is always for the legs to lift unless the trunk is bent. Bending the trunk reduces the effect of leverage, and makes the trunk 'lighter'.

As an example of this mechanism, study fig. 31. Two boys are sitting on a seesaw. The one on the right weighs 22 kg (50 lb), but the boy on the left is heavier and weighs 27 kg (60 lb). The seesaw is balanced at the moment, but if the lighter boy wants to lift the heavier boy, the heavier boy must move closer to the pivot point. This reduces his leverage effect and can be thought of as making him 'lighter'.

The same principle applies with the sit-up. If the trunk is to lift instead of the legs, the leverage effect of the trunk must be reduced. To do this the trunk must bend so that its weight moves closer to the hip which is acting as the pivot in this

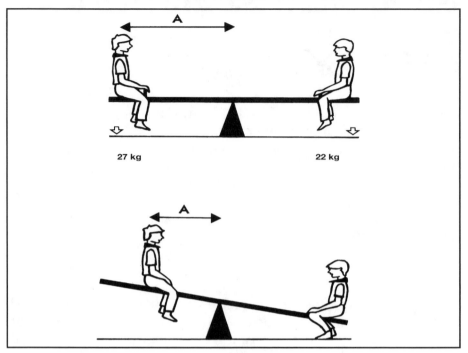

Fig. 31 *Leverage: 'A' is the length of the lever which the heavier boy is using*

exercise (*see* fig. 32). If you are able to bend your trunk sufficiently, you will be able to sit up. But, if your abdominal muscles are weak or lengthened, your trunk will not bend enough to reduce its leverage, and so your trunk will stay on the ground and your legs will lift instead.

The abdominal muscles work to bend the trunk, but the lifting action which pulls the trunk away from the floor is carried out

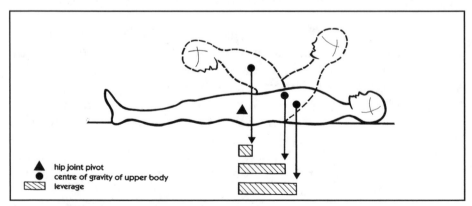

▲ hip joint pivot
● centre of gravity of upper body
▨ leverage

Fig. 32 *Changing leverage in a sit-up*

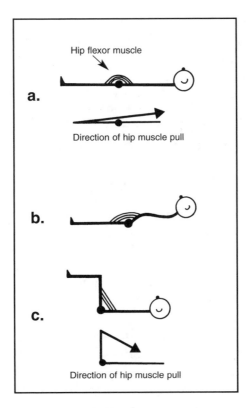

Fig. 33 (a) In the lying position the hip flexors pull parallel to the spine causing little lifting effect but maximal spinal compression; (b) when the hip flexors pull they can arch the spine; (c) bending the knees reduces spinal compression

by the hip flexor muscles. These will pull hard on the spine to try to lift it up. If the legs are straight, the hip flexor muscles lie almost parallel to the spine (see fig. 33a). The muscles find it very difficult to lift the spine from this position, and instead they pull the lower spine into an arched position (see fig. 33b). If the knees and hips are bent (see fig. 33c), the hip flexor muscles are lifted up and they can now move the spine more easily and as a result will compress it less. Bending the hip therefore considerably reduces the stress on the lumbar spine.

● ● ● ● ● ● ● ● ● ● ● ● ● ● ● **KEYPOINT** ● ● ● ● ● ● ● ● ● ● ● ● ● ●
Bending the legs in a sit-up reduces the unwanted forces on the lower back.

It must be emphasised that the stress on the spine from hip flexor action only occurs because the trunk is lifted clear of the ground. The action of lifting the trunk rather than simply curling it does not increase the work of the abdominals substantially, and is really unnecessary from the point of view of abdominal training. If the trunk stays on the ground, with the abdominals being used to bend the trunk only, the effects on the lumbar spine are reduced once again and the exercise becomes quite safe. This is why in the F.L.A.T. programme we use the trunk curl instead of the standard sit-up. It is more effective and far safer.

Fixing the feet during a sit-up enables you to pull harder with the hip flexor muscles. This in turn can increase the stress on the spine, and allow you to sit up without needing to bend your spine. The effect is therefore to increase the work of the hip flexors but reduce the work of the abdominals, precisely opposite to what we require from the exercise. In this programme we do not use foot fixation for basic abdominal exercises.

Inclining the sit-up bench changes the leverage effect on the spine (*see* fig. 34). In a normal sit-up (*see* fig. 34a) performed from the floor, the leverage acting on the trunk is maximum at the beginning of the exercise. As the trunk lifts, the leverage

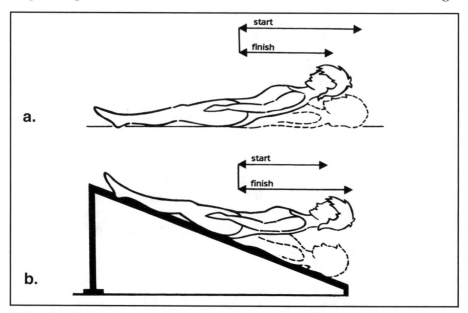

Fig. 34 *The inclined sit-up: (a) leverage reduces as movement continues; (b) leverage increases up to the mid-point of the movement*

reduces. If we incline the sit-up bench, however (*see* fig. 34b), the leverage lessens at the beginning of the movement but increases to its maximum about halfway through the exercise as the body moves into the horizontal position. As the trunk lifts further, it moves away from the horizontal and so the leverage forces reduce again. Inclining the bench makes the exercise harder therefore.

THE LEG RAISE ●

The leg raise can in some ways be seen as the reverse of the sit-up. With this exercise, the trunk stays on the ground and the legs are lifted instead. The movement now is purely from the hip flexors. They work to pull the legs up from the ground. However, again because the hip flexors lie parallel with the spine, they will tend to arch the lumbar spine and subject it to forces large enough to damage it severely. The problem occurs because as well as attaching to the lumbar spine, the hip flexors attach to the pelvis. As they pull, they will tend to tip the pelvis and pull the lumbar spine out of alignment. Normally the abdominal muscles will contract to stop this unwanted action occurring (*see* fig. 35a). If they are weak, however, the abdominals will be unable to do this and the pelvis will tilt, placing stress on the lumbar spine (*see* fig. 35b).

The problem can be greatly reduced if the legs are bent to reduce their leverage effect (*see* fig. 35c). The reduced leverage means that the abdominal muscles do not have to work as hard to hold the pelvis and lumbar spine in place. If they are weak, the abdominals may only be able to hold the pelvis still against the reduced leverage of the bent legs. In addition, if the hips are bent, the hip flexors can now pull at an angle rather than parallel to the spine. They will therefore compress the spine less, and be more effective in creating hip movement instead.

Leverage forces applied from the legs are greatest when the leg is horizontal. When performing this exercise, therefore, we must keep the legs away from the horizontal. This can be achieved by performing the exercise against a wall with the legs beginning vertical. As the legs lower, the pelvis must be kept still. If it begins to tip, the exercise should stop because the abdominal muscles are failing to hold the pelvis stable. At this point, the legs are rested against the wall to take the weight off the spine. The movement is now to lower the legs from the vertical towards the wall rather than raising them from the floor.

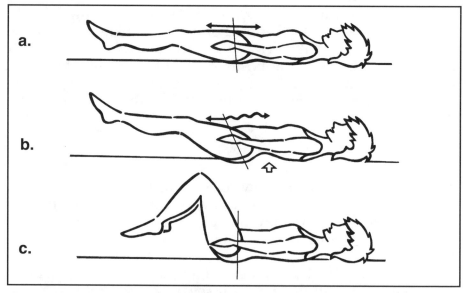

Fig. 35 *The leg raise: (a) as the hip flexor muscles pull on the pelvis, the abdominals stop the pelvis from tilting; (b) if the abdominals are weak, the pelvis tips forward, hollowing the lower back as the legs are lifted; (c) bending the knees reduces the leverage effect*

The same reservation applies with this exercise as with the sit-up. The hip flexors are working primarily, and the abdominals are holding the spine still. If we want to work the abdominals harder, we must modify the leg raise so that the spine bends and the tail lifts off the ground. This exercise is the 'pelvic raise', sometimes called the 'reverse crunch'. It is described on page 102 and forms an essential part of the F.L.A.T. programme.

• • • • • • • • • • • • • • • **KEYPOINT** • • • • • • • • • • • • • • • •
Do not allow the legs to move into a horizontal position when performing a leg raise action.

THE TRUNK CRUNCH •

The trunk crunch is a modification of the standard sit-up originally used by professional bodybuilders. As such it is an intense exercise and not suitable for the novice.

The exercise begins lying on the floor on your back. The knees and hips are bent to 90°, and the calves are placed on a bench or chair. From this position a sit-up is performed, moving the head towards the knees.

The exercise begins in the same way as the sit-up, with the abdominal muscles working hard. Because the pelvis remains still, the emphasis of the exercise is on the upper abdominals with the lower portion of the muscles showing less activity. As the spine bends maximally you reach a point where you must lift yourself up from the floor. In lighter subjects this may not be possible, but those who have heavier legs will be able to achieve this movement. Performing the action with the legs fixed enables you to pull the feet against the fixation point. As this happens the hip flexor muscles pull hard to lift the spine off the ground.

If the action is performed with a twist, the oblique abdominals will work more, but the central abdominal muscle (rectus abdominis) will still work hard.

Although a useful exercise because it strongly emphasises the upper portion of the abdominal muscles, it must be balanced out by using the pelvic raise to work the lower portion of the muscles. Failure to do this will leave an imbalance between the upper and lower portion of the abdominals, a situation which could lead to back pain.

The trunk crunch is not suitable for those who have suffered from back pain or those who require light training. It is included as an advanced exercise in the F.L.A.T. programme, performed with the feet not fixed to reduce stress on the lower spine. In the programme, use of the exercise is balanced by performing the pelvic raise in the same exercise session.

> •••••••••••••••• **KEYPOINT** ••••••••••••••••
> The trunk crunch is an advanced exercise to be used only
> after initial abdominal strength has been gained using other
> exercises. The crunch focuses on the upper abdominal region,
> and must be balanced by movements which emphasise the
> lower abdominal area, such as the pelvic raise.

THE KNEE RAISE (HIP FLEXOR) •••••••••••••••••••

The hip flexor station is a standard attachment to many multigym weight training units and is often found in many commercial gym set-ups. The machine consists of a back pad and two side gutter pads to take the forearms.

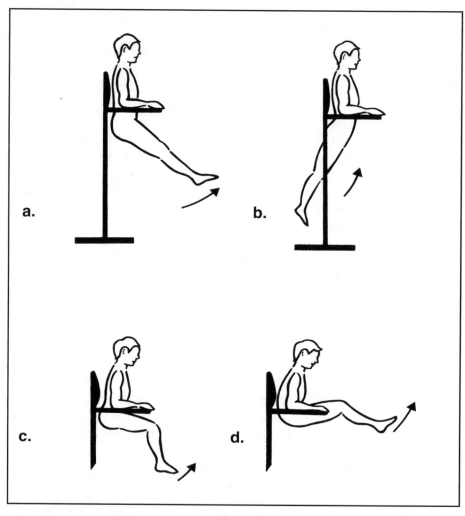

Fig. 36 *The knee raise: (a) the abdominals work to hold the pelvis firm at the beginning of the movement; (b) if the legs are allowed to swing backwards, the lower back will hollow dangerously (hyper-extend); (c) knees and hips bent to 90°; (d) trunk flexes to lift legs*

Normal instructions are to lift yourself up into the machine with your elbows bent to 90° and your forearms in the gutter pads (*see* fig. 36). The small of your back is pressed against the back pad. From this position lift your legs, keeping them straight, to the horizontal position and then lower them down again.

As the legs lift, the hip flexors work. To stabilise the spine and pelvis the abdominal muscles tighten. Only when the spine begins to bend, as the legs near the horizontal position, do the abdominals work to actively bend the spine. Although the exercise feels hard, the greatest amount of the work is from the hip flexors, with the abdominals receiving only a poor workout.

One of the major problems with this exercise stems from the length of the hamstring muscles on the back of the thigh. In many people these muscles are very short. When this is the case, you are not able to lift the legs out straight without the knees bending. If you try to hold the knees straight, the tight hamstrings will pull on the pelvis and cause the lower spine to bend. This can place stress on the spine.

A second area of concern is due to momentum. Because some people find the exercise hard, there is a tendency to swing the legs to assist the movement. When this happens, the momentum of the heavy legs moving at speed becomes uncontrollable. As the legs are lowered, they swing backwards forcing the back to hyperextend (*see* fig. 36b) and severely stressing the spine.

The hip flexor exercise can be made safer and more effective with some modifications. Firstly, the knees should be bent to relax the hamstrings and so reduce the stress on the lower back. In addition, bending the knees reduces the leverage effect and makes the exercise more controllable. If the knees are bent to 90° and kept still, the action can then be one of bending the trunk to pull the tailbone away from the pad (*see* fig. 36c). This increases the emphasis on the abdominal muscles, making the exercise more effective. Secondly, any swinging of the legs should be avoided. As the legs are lowered they should be under control. In the bottom position, pause before you start to lift the legs again. In this way momentum is cut down and the back is not forced into an unnatural position.

• • • • • • • • • • • • • • • **KEYPOINT** • • • • • • • • • • • • • • • •
The knee raise can place stress on the lower back if it is performed with a 'swinging' action. Keep the action under control at all times, especially when lowering the legs.

TRUNK EXERCISE DANGERS

More than any other area in the body, the back is susceptible to injury through incorrect exercise. To prevent injury, we need to have an understanding of some basic mechanical concepts.

LEVERAGE

The limbs and spine act as levers when we move. A lever is simply a rigid bar which moves around a fixed point or pivot. Two forces act on the lever: effort and resistance. The effort tries to move the lever, while the resistance tries to stop movement. In the body, the effort is supplied by your muscles, while the resistance is the weight of the body part. Take as an example the leg lifting from a lying position. The pivot is the hip joint, the effort is supplied by the hip flexor muscles which lift the leg, and the resistance is the weight of the whole leg. The effort from the muscle acts at the point where the muscle attaches to the thighbone (*see* fig. 37b).

We say that the weight acts through a single point called the 'centre of gravity'. This is really the balance point of the limb, and would be the centre point of the limb if the limb were the same size all over. However, because the leg is thicker at the top, the centre of gravity lies towards the heavier end.

Leverage is greater when there is a long horizontal distance between the pivot and the point where the weight or effort acts. In the example above, the leverage is greatest when the leg first lifts from the ground, because it is close to the horizontal. As the leg lifts up, it moves away from the horizontal and so the leverage reduces and the exercise actually gets easier. In fig. 37c the subject is standing up with the legs in the vertical position. The leverage to begin with is minimal. As the leg lifts, however, it moves towards the horizontal and so the leverage increases. This is now the reverse situation to fig. 37a, and the exercise gradually gets harder. Although both exercises involve flexing the straight leg, the starting position of the movement changes the effect of the exercise considerably.

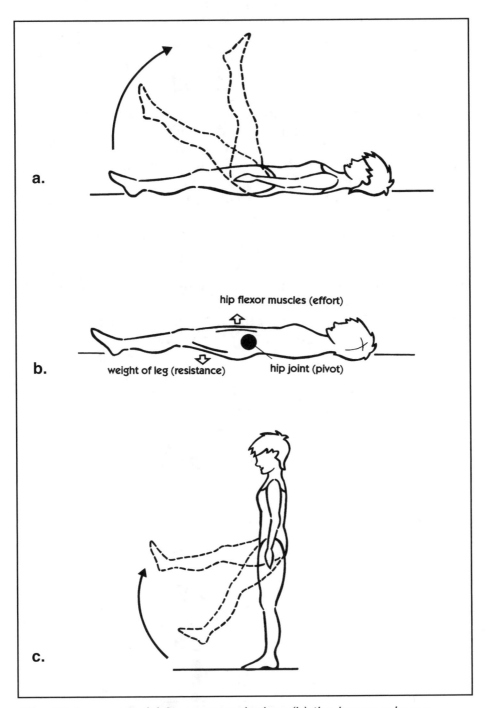

Fig. 37 *Leverage: (a) leverage reducing; (b) the leg as a lever; (c) leverage increasing*

> •••••••••••••••• *KEYPOINT* ••••••••••••••••••
> Leverage is greatest when a lever is in a horizontal position.

This example has important implications with regard to the safety of the spine. Exercises which involve moving the spine into a horizontal position will place great amounts of leverage on the spine and should be used with caution. Often, simply altering the starting position will move the spine away from the horizontal and so reduce the stress on the lower back. Where a horizontal position must be used, the spine should be supported. As an example of this process let's look at a common stretch for the hamstring muscles on the back of the thigh. In fig. 38a an athlete is stretching the hamstrings by bending the trunk forwards from the hip. This action places an excessive leverage stress on the spine because it is moving from a vertical position (minimal leverage) to a more horizontal position (maximum leverage). Simply by placing one hand down on the knee, the spine is supported and the stress reduced (*see* fig. 38b).

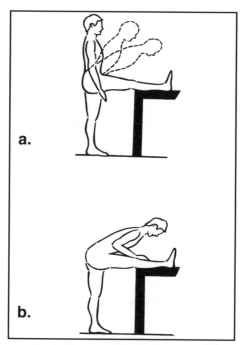

Fig. 38 *Supporting the body when leverage is large: (a) spine moves towards the horizontal, leverage increases; (b) bodyweight taken through the arm at the point of maximum leverage*

••••••••••••••••• *KEYPOINT* •••••••••••••••••
If an exercise doesn't allow you to keep your spine vertical,
place your hand on something for support.

WHICH BODY AREA IS MOVING? • • • • • • • • • • • • • • • •

Often, a quick look at an exercise creates the impression that a particular part of the body is moving. On closer inspection, however, it can be seen that other body areas are also moving and these may be taking greater stress than was intended. This holds true particularly with the pelvis moving on the spine or hip. Take as an example a stretch for the thigh muscles (*see* fig. 39). The subject is standing up straight and has grasped the ankle. They are pulling the hip backwards and trying to increase the bend on the knee at the same time. At first sight this seems to be an exercise which is simply placing the thigh muscles into a stretch. However, if we look closely we can see that the pelvis has tilted forwards and stress is now placed on the spine. In this case the spine is more flexible than the tight thigh muscles, so the more the stretch is pushed, the more stress is thrown on to the spine.

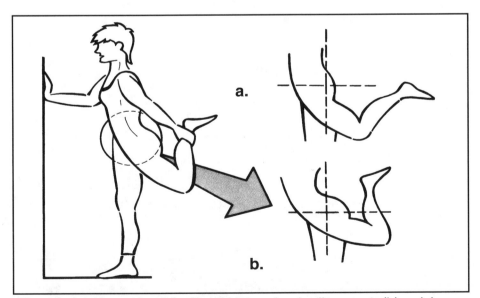

Fig. 39 (a) Normal pelvic tilt and lower back alignment; (b) pelvis moves excessively, causing lower back to hollow: leg goes higher, but technique is faulty

If we look at fig. 40, the subjects are trying to touch their toes by stretching their hamstrings (behind the thigh). The subject in fig. 40b appears to be stretching further because they have reached closer to their toes. However, if we look at the line of the pelvis, both individuals have moved exactly the same amount. The extra movement in fig. 40b has occurred by overbending the upper spine. Again, this part of the body is generally more flexible than the tight hamstrings. As the movement is pushed further and further, the stretch on the hamstrings will not increase, but the stress on the upper spine certainly will.

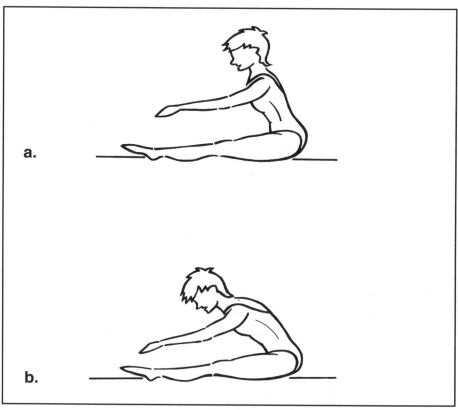

Fig. 40 *(a) Normal movement; (b) excessive movement of upper spine*

●●●●●●●●●●●●●● **KEYPOINT** ●●●●●●●●●●●●●●
Looking at the pelvis gives an important indication of lumbar spine position.

MOMENTUM •

Momentum is a combination of how heavy an object is and how quickly it is moving. A heavy object, such as the leg or trunk, which is moving quickly, will possess a great deal of momentum and will be very difficult to stop. The high momentum can take over the movement, and you may find that you are no longer able to control a body part. This is when injuries can occur.

There are two methods to make this type of exercise safer. Firstly, you can reduce the momentum by slowing the movement down where heavy body parts are used. In the programme, all movements of the trunk are slow to begin with. It is only when we have a considerable degree of control over an action that speed is increased.

The second way to make a movement safer, if it is moving quickly, is to ensure that the movement only occurs in the middle of the joint range. The joint range is the total movement from one extreme to the other (*see* page 8). In the case of the knee, it would be from the fully bent position to fully straight. Where an action is rapid, we must restrict the movement to the middle part of this range so that the joint is never fully bent or fully straightened. In this way we reduce the likelihood of injuring the joint tissues by overstretching them.

> • • • • • • • • • • • • • • • **KEYPOINT** • • • • • • • • • • • • • • • •
> Keep movements slow and controlled. Use the middle of a
> joint's total movement more often than the ends.

EXCESSIVE LUMBAR CURVATURE • • • • • • • • • • • • • • • • •

We have seen earlier that pelvic tilt is intimately linked with lumbar curvature. Tilting the pelvis forwards increases the lumbar curve, while tilting it backwards flattens it. One of the aims of this programme is to enable a subject to identify the neutral position of the spine, where the pelvis is level, and to hold this position while performing other movements.

If the pelvis is allowed to tilt too far, the lumbar spine will move to its end point. At this point the disc, spinal facet joints and lumbar tissues are all stressed excessively. Increasing the curve will press the facet joints together, while flattening the curve will push the spinal disc backwards. In each case the ligaments surrounding the spinal tissues are overstretched.

A number of abdominal exercises will tend to increase the lumbar curve dangerously. In the straight leg raise action (*see* fig. 41a), the pull of the hip muscles on to the pelvis and lumbar spine tends to tilt the pelvis forwards and lift the lumbar spine away from the ground. Even if the spine remains flat on the floor, the hip muscles still pull dangerously hard on to the lower spine, compressing the discs and increasing the likelihood of injury. The safer alternative to this exercise is the heel slide (*see* page 93). Now only one leg is lifting at a time, the other one remaining on the floor to provide support and increase stability. In addition, the heel of the leg which moves stays on the ground so the full weight is not lifted.

With spinal hyperextension exercises in an unsupported position (*see* fig. 41b), the abdominal muscles may be unable to support the spine and hold it in its neutral position. As a consequence the pelvis tilts forwards and the lumbar spine moves too far into extension. As we have seen, this position compresses the joints in the base of the spine. This compression is compounded by the powerful contraction of the spinal extensor muscles which are fighting to hold the body up. Alternatives to this exercise include bridging (*see* page 106) and the spinal extension hold (*see* page 124). In each case the whole bodyweight is not taken until all the trunk muscles are strong enough to do this. When the muscles are strong, the pelvis is aligned and the abdominal hollowing procedure is practised first, before the exercise begins. In this way the spine is correctly aligned before it is loaded.

Overhead pressing actions in weight training can also lead to hyperextension of the lumbar spine through the pelvis tilt mechanism if the abdominal muscles fail to contract at the onset of the lift (*see* fig. 41c). To prevent this happening, firstly the abdominal hollowing procedure must be practised throughout the lift. Secondly, the limiting factor should not be the amount of weight that can be lifted overhead, but the point at which the pelvis begins to tilt. When this happens, the exercise must stop, however large or small the weight being lifted.

Flattening of the lumbar spine is common in sitting positions. Squatting on to a bench which is too low, for example (*see* fig. 41d), will allow the pelvis to tilt backwards and this in turn pulls the spinal bones into a flexed position. Done at speed, this type of action can be extremely dangerous. The movement can be modified in two ways. Firstly, the bench height must be adjusted so that it is just higher than the subject's knee. In this way the amount of knee and hip movement is reduced and the lumbar spine will not be rounded as far. Secondly, the movement should be slowed down so that the momentum is reduced. In this way, less stress is passed on to the spine, and the action stays controlled all the time.

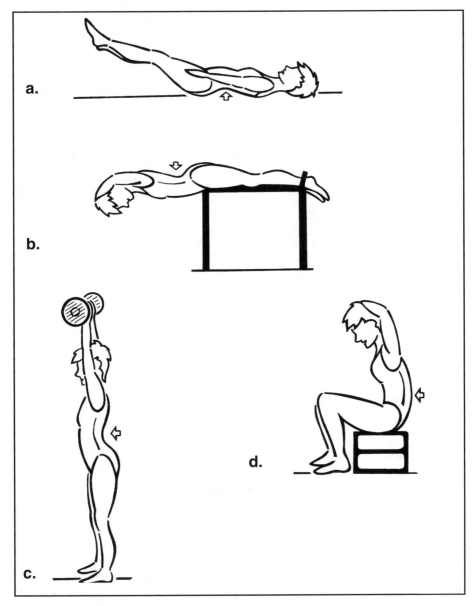

Fig. 41 Excessive lumbar curvature

•••••••••••••••••• **KEYPOINT** •••••••••••••••••••
Try to keep your spine in the neutral position as often as
possible.

NECK POSTURE •

In an earlier section we saw that the posture line can be used to
determine optimal posture. With reference to the head and neck,
the posture line should pass through the shoulder joint and also
through the ear. A common faulty alignment seen in exercise is
where the head is held forward (*see* fig. 42a). The ear can be seen
to move about 5–10 cm (2–4 in.) forwards of the posture line and
well in front of the shoulder. This stresses the neck tissues and is
very dangerous when performed at speed. The movement is
common when the head is used to lead, and provides
momentum to get an action started. This is especially true of sit-
up-type exercises. If a subject is attempting to sit up from the
ground, they may be unable to do so if their abdominal muscles
are very weak. One way that they can cover this up is to perform
the action quickly and use the weight of the head to 'fling' the
body off the ground (*see* fig. 42b). This rapid action can damage
the neck structures sufficiently to cause a trapped nerve and
even a type of whiplash injury.

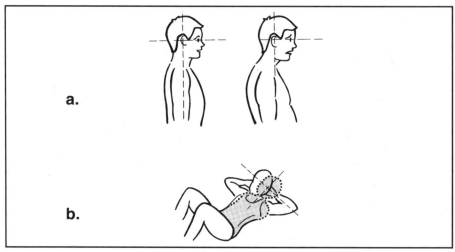

Fig. 42 *Neck position: (a) correct (left); too far forward (right);*
(b) placing the hands behind the head during a sit-up forces the
head forwards and stresses the neck. The dotted figure shows the
correct alignment

To avoid this neck posture, the chin should be held back, in alignment with the rest of the spine. This position is held so the head does not move, and the action is performed slowly, under control.

• • • • • • • • • • • • • • • • *KEYPOINT* • • • • • • • • • • • • • • • • •
Avoid nodding your head when performing abdominal exercises.

STABILITY •

Three factors are important to stability: the size and alignment of the base of support, and the centre of gravity. An object's base of support is the total area that is on the ground or, in the case of the human body, the distance between the feet (*see* fig. 43). If the base of support is wide, the weight of the object is distributed over a large area and the object is therefore stable, like a pyramid. When the base of support is small, as with a ballet dancer *en point*, the object is unstable and likely to wobble off balance. When choosing an exercise position, therefore, we should make sure that our base of support is as wide as is comfortable.

The second factor concerning the base of support which is important to stability is the direction in which it faces. Aligning your feet so that they face the way you are moving makes you more stable. For example, if you have your feet one in front of the other, although your base of support is large, you will still be unstable if you are practising a side bend movement. This is because the side bend movement occurs in a side-to-side direction, but your feet position has widened your base of support in a forward-to-back direction. To be stable while performing side bends your feet must be apart in a sideways direction. Similarly, if your feet are apart sideways you are unstable when performing shoulder rounding and bracing. This movement occurs front-to-back, so your base of support should be widened in this direction.

The third factor which is important to stability is the height of your bodyweight above the ground. When you stand tall, you are less stable and there is a tendency to topple when performing exercises. Simply bending your knees lowers your bodyweight closer to the ground and makes you more stable.

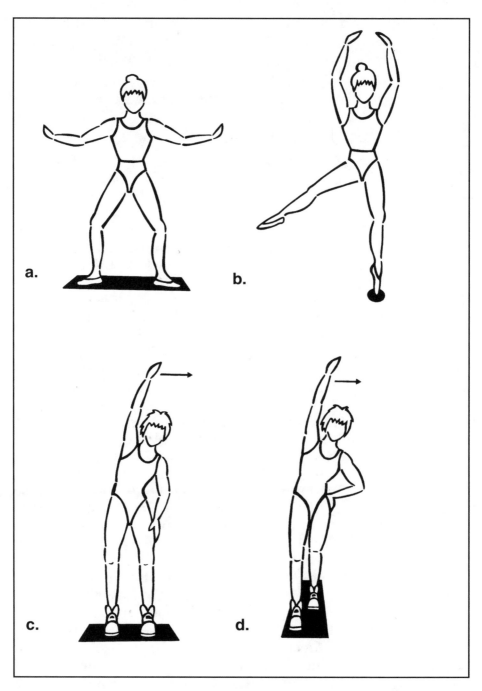

Fig. 43 *Stability: (a) black area is the base of support – stable when wide; (b) unstable – small base of support; (c) base is wide in direction of movement – stable; (d) base is widened in direction different to movement – less stable*

```
• • • • • • • • • • • • • • • • KEYPOINT • • • • • • • • • • • • • • • • • •
To make yourself more stable, keep your feet apart and face
the direction of travel. Bend your knees slightly.
```

COMFORT

An exercise which is uncomfortable can also be dangerous. When you are not comfortable you tend to alter your posture regularly, and wriggle. This takes concentration away from the exercise and affects stability. An exercise usually becomes uncomfortable if you are placing weight through a bony point such as the knee, hip or tailbone, and pressure builds up. In each of these cases try to rest the body part on a mat or folded towel instead of on the floor alone.

Taking up an unnatural posture will also make you uncomfortable as it will stress the body tissues excessively. When using equipment, therefore, make sure it is adjusted to suit your body size. This is especially true of weight training apparatus where correct seat height adjustment is vital to allow correct spinal alignment.

SUMMARY

• The centre of gravity of an object is its balance point.
• In a lever, the further away from the pivot a weight is placed, the greater the leverage effect.
• Momentum is a combination of how heavy an object is and how fast it is moving.
• Tilting the pelvis forwards *increases* the lumbar curve; tilting it backwards *decreases* it.
• Stability is determined by the size and alignment of an object's base of support and the position of its centre of gravity.

Before we start

Preparation ●

Before we begin exercising we need to consider a few things in preparation.

The body takes time to change from its resting 'tick-over' to a point where it is ready to face the rigours of intense exercise. Just as a car needs to be warmed up before it will run smoothly, so the body must speed up gradually to be at its best. When you are cold, your body tissues are stiffer and less pliable. This means that your joints and muscles can be damaged more easily. In order to reduce the likelihood of injury and make exercise more effective, we need to practise a warm-up.

A warm-up can either be 'passive', where the body is heated from the outside, or 'active', where exercise is used to form the heat internally. An example of a passive warm-up is to have a hot shower or sauna, while an active warm-up can be achieved by gentle jogging, for example. Both types of warm-up can be effective, but are appropriate to different situations. An active warm-up is the type normally used before general exercise, while a passive warm-up is useful when you may be recovering from an injury, and it would not be safe to practise vigorous exercise.

To be effective, a warm-up should be intense enough to cause mild sweating. Gentle jogging, light aerobics, or cycling on an exercise bicycle, are all good warm-up activities. These types of movements are known as *pulse raising* exercises and should make you breathe faster and more deeply than usual, raising your pulse rate comfortably. The activities should challenge the body but not exhaust it: aim to be able to carry out a normal conversation when you are using pulse raising exercise – you should not be so out of breath that you find it hard to speak. The joints should be taken through their full range of movement, starting with small movements, gradually becoming larger. Slowly circle the arms, twist the spine, and bend the legs until all the major joints have been worked. The emphasis is on slow, controlled movements which do not stress the body, but which prepare it for activity. These movements are known as *mobility* exercises, because they aim to move all the major joints, helping to lubricate them and making movements smoother and more flowing. Mobility exercises are different from the stretching exercises used on pages 43–9 in connection with posture. For mobility exercises the aim is to take the joints through their full movement range *as part of* the warm-up: with stretching we are actually trying to increase the movement range and so need to be *thoroughly warmed up* beforehand.

For skilled movements, such as those used in the F.L.A.T. programme, an additional function of the warm-up is *rehearsal*. In other words, the warm-up movements should actually practise any basic skills that are to be used in the main exercise programme. For all the F.L.A.T. exercises two movements are vital:

- finding and maintaining the *neutral position*
- activating the deep corset muscles in a *hollowing* (abdominal pulling-in) action

and the two exercises which rehearse these actions are pelvic tilting (page 84) and abdominal hollowing (page 89). These two actions should therefore be used as part of a warm up.

A WARM-UP FOR ABDOMINAL TRAINING

As with all other exercise programmes, a warm-up is required before beginning the F.L.A.T. programme. The foundation movements by their nature are very gentle and may themselves be used as part of a warm-up.

Aim to mobilise the hips, spine and shoulders, raise the pulse rate, and rehearse the neutral and hollowing position (*see* fig. 43).

- **Shoulders**: hold on to a towel and simply reach overhead keeping the arms straight. Do not arch the back while doing this, and make sure that the movement is slow and controlled.
- **Spine**: flexion (rounding) and extension (hollowing) is carried out at the same time as rehearsing the neutral position, both movements using the pelvic tilt. Tilt the pelvis backwards and then forwards five times and stop at the mid-position, with the lumbar spine slightly hollow – this is the neutral position.
- **Rotation**: slowly turn so that you look to the right and then to the left, gently twisting the whole of the spine, including the neck, thoracic spine (chest level) and lumbar spine (lower back). Again the action should be slow and controlled.
- **Side bending**: rest the hands slightly below the hips, at mid-thigh level. Use the hands for support and slowly bend to the right and then stand straight again. Repeat the action to the left.

Aim	Action
• Mobility of shoulders, hips and spine	• Overhead reach – 10 reps • Flexion–extension of lumbar spine with pelvic tilt (*see* below) • Rotation of lumbar spine – 5 reps to each side • Side bending of lumbar spine – 5 reps to each side • Knee lifts – 5 reps each knee
• Raise pulse rate	• Static cycle or brisk walking in well-padded shoes – 2–5 mins
• Rehearse foundation actions	• Pelvic tilt, standing (page 84) – 3 reps • Abdominal hollowing, standing (page 89) – 3 reps

Fig. 43 The abdominal training warm-up

• **Hip mobility**: hold on to the back of a chair and raise one knee as far a you can towards the chest, bending at both the knee and the hip. Make sure you keep standing straight and do not bend your spine.

The pulse raising activity may be a brisk walk (wear well-padded shoes to minimise jarring) or a cycle on a static bike in the gym, for example. Before you perform any specific abdominal exercises remind yourself of the abdominal hollowing action (page 89) by performing this three times, taking care not be move the spine and to breath normally (don't hold your breath or take a deep breath).

COMFORT •

Clothing should be warm to maintain body heat, and loose-fitting to allow unrestricted movement. Shorts and a T-shirt are fine for warmer weather, but fleecy jogging bottoms and a sweatshirt are normally better when it is cooler. Remember that you may need to see your spine in the mirror at some stage of the exercise programme, so try to wear layers of clothing which you can gradually remove.

Make sure that you can move without restriction from furniture or other people. A little time spent clearing some space in the room you are going to exercise in is well worthwhile. You may need a small exercise mat or a number of folded towels to hand for padding during exercises where you are kneeling or lying on the floor.

> • • • • • • • • • • • • • • • • **KEYPOINT** • • • • • • • • • • • • • • • • •
> Wear comfortable clothing, and warm up gradually before you
> begin the F.L.A.T. programme.

Following exercise, you will need to warm down by reducing your activity slowly, rather than with a sudden jolt. This will have the additional benefit of reducing muscle ache.

FOUNDATION

We begin the programme by mastering two essential movements. These form the cornerstones of F.L.A.T. and are often used as parts of other more advanced exercises later in the programme. The foundation movements are important because they involve re-learning important skills relating to control of spinal movement which have often been forgotten. Were you to try to perform abdominal exercises before you have mastered these skills, your movement control would be so poor that injury may result. Time spent on the foundation exercises is therefore a sound investment for the future.

Because the foundation movements are practising *skills*, they should be used regularly throughout the day rather than simply during an exercise programme.

PELVIC TILTING

We saw on page 9 that the tilt of the pelvis determines the position of the lower back. Tilting the pelvis forwards increases the hollow in the small of the back, while tilting the pelvis backwards flattens the back, reducing the lumbar hollow. The reason pelvic tilting is so important is that it teaches control of the lumbar spine during exercise. An incorrect pelvic tilt during exercise can lead to excessive movement in the lower spine. We must be able to identify this when it is happening, by feeling the action taking place, so that we can correct it before an injury occurs. Because accurate control of this action is so vital, we practise the movement from two different starting positions.

PELVIC TILTING, LYING

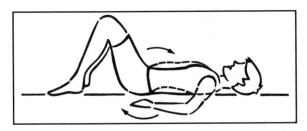

■ Starting position
Begin lying on your back with your knees bent. Place your feet and knees shoulder width apart. Your arms should rest on the floor slightly away from your body.

■ Action
Tighten your abdominal muscles and your buttock muscles to tip your pelvis backwards and flatten the small of your back against the floor. Pause and then reverse the action, tightening your back and hip muscles to hollow the small of your back away from the floor. Repeat this action and try to stop the movement when you are halfway between the two extremes. *This mid-point is your neutral position.*

■ Points to note
The pelvic tilting action should be brought about by contraction of the abdominal muscles and buttock muscles together. Although it is possible to perform the action with one set of muscles alone, working both sets will give you more control.

■ Training tip
The action must be smooth and controlled rather than jerky. A jerking action will stress the lower spine.

PELVIC TILTING, STANDING

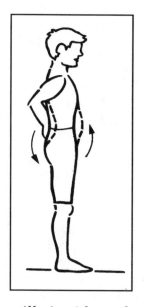

■ Starting position
Begin standing with your feet shoulder width apart, arms by your sides. Stand tall. Do not slouch.

■ Action
Tighten your abdominal muscles and your buttock muscles together to tilt your pelvis backwards and flatten your lower spine. Pause and then tighten your hips and spinal muscles to increase the hollow in the small of your back.

■ Points to note
The action should be isolated to your lower back. Your shoulders should stay square, and your knees should remain still. Avoid any body sway.

■ Training tip
Placing your hands out to the side in a 'T' shape will help with the balance of this exercise, and make any unwanted body sway more obvious.

PELVIC TILTING, ON A GYM BALL

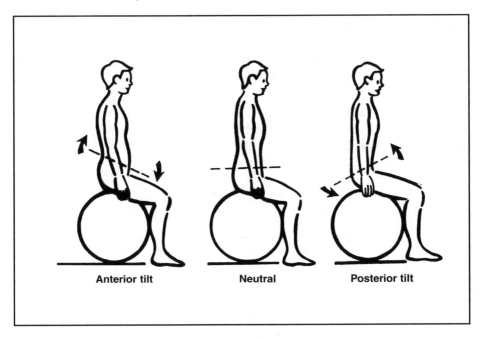

Anterior tilt   Neutral   Posterior tilt

■ Starting position
Sit on a large 60 cm (24 in.) gym ball with your knees bent to 90°. Your back should be straight but not rigid, and your feet should be flat on the floor.

■ Action
Draw your tummy in (abdominal hollow) and then tilt your pelvis forwards to increase the hollow in the small of your back, and then backwards to decrease it.

■ Points to note
The movement must be isolated to the pelvis. Do not allow any body sway and do not round or brace your shoulders.

■ Training tip
To prevent body sway to begin with, place a dining chair at each side of the ball. Put each hand flat on the chair surfaces to monitor shoulder movement.

ABDOMINAL HOLLOWING • • • • • • • • • • • • • • • • • •

We saw on pages 13 and 15 that the transversus abdominis is an important muscle to maintain stability of the lower spine. This muscle is often not used in exercise programmes, but it is vital that we work it before we move on to further abdominal training. The muscle works hard during the abdominal hollowing actions described below. Even if you have been training for many years, practise this movement because you may be surprised at just how little control you have in this body area.

ABDOMINAL HOLLOWING, KNEELING

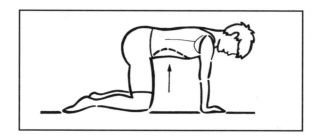

■ Starting position
Begin kneeling on all fours with your hands and knees shoulder width apart. Kneel on a mat or folded towel for comfort.

■ Action
Allow your tummy muscles to relax and sag downwards to the floor. Then tighten them and pull them up and in, trying to hollow your tummy.

■ Points to note
Initially the amount of movement may be very small, but with practice you should notice 10–15 cm (4–6 in.) of movement in total. Breathe normally throughout the action; do not take a deep breath when trying to flatten your tummy. Keep your spine still as you hollow. Do not arch the spine or tilt the pelvis.

■ Training tip
Place a mirror on the floor beneath your tummy so you can see what is happening. Focus your attention on your tummy button, and try to move it rather than the whole of your abdomen.

ABDOMINAL HOLLOWING, LYING

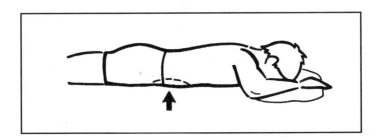

■ Starting position
Lie on the floor on a mat or towel with your arms either by your sides or folded forwards. Keep your feet comfortably apart, and place a folded towel beneath your forehead to avoid squashing your nose.

■ Action
Perform the abdominal hollowing action by pulling your tummy button inwards and drawing your abdominal wall (tummy surface) off the floor.

■ Points to note
If your are a little overweight and have a little bit of a 'pot belly', you may not be able to do this exercise! Make sure that you draw your tummy off the floor just with abdominal muscle action; do not take a deep breath or lift your chest.

■ Training tip
Train with a partner and lie on a hand towel placed under your tummy. As you pull the muscles in tight in the hollowing action, your partner should be able to pull the towel sideways.

ABDOMINAL HOLLOWING, SITTING

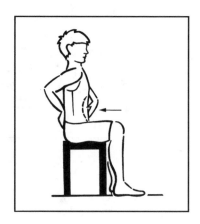

■ Starting position
Sit on a stool with your knees apart. Sit tall with your back slightly hollow. Place one hand on your tummy and the other in the small of your back.

■ Action
Perform the abdominal hollowing action by pulling your tummy in and up away from your front hand, focusing your attention on your tummy button.

■ Points to note
When sitting, try to sit tall, rather than slouching or holding the trunk too rigid.

■ Training tip
Use your hands to monitor the neutral position of your spine and also to give you feedback about the abdominal hollowing action.

ABDOMINAL HOLLOWING, STANDING

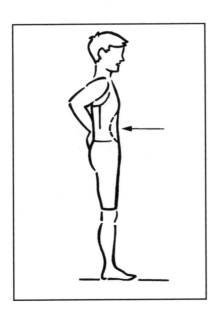

■ Starting position
Stand upright with your feet shoulder width apart. Place your lower spine in its neutral position.

■ Action
Perform the abdominal hollowing action by focusing on your tummy button and pulling it in and up.

■ Points to note
Breathe normally throughout the movement; do not hold your breath. Make sure that your spine, hips and legs stay still. Isolate the movement to your tummy alone; do not flatten your back or tilt your pelvis.

■ Training tip
Begin by practising this exercise standing side-on to a mirror. Place a belt loosely around your lower tummy. As you hollow, a gap should form between your tummy and the belt.

COMMON MISTAKES •

There are several mistakes which you must take care not to make when performing the abdominal hollowing action. These are outlined in fig. 44.

Mistake	Noticeable by	Reason	How to correct
Rib cage rises	Look at the base of the ribs just above the umbilicus. This should remain on a horizontal line	Subject has taken a deep breath	Place your finger-tips on the subject's lower ribs and encourage them to hollow the abdomen while keeping their ribs on your fingers. Instruct the subject to breath normally
Rib cage depresses	Base of rib cage moves downwards	Subject has activated the rectus abdominis and external oblique muscles	Encourage the subject to put less effort into the hollowing action and to begin the contraction by tightening the pelvic floor
Spine flexes	Back bends and head comes forwards	Subject has activated the rectus abdominis muscle and lost body alignment	Ask the subject to perform the hollowing action while standing with their back against the wall
Breath held	Colour changes of face, subject becomes breathless	Subject is not able to dissociate breathing from abdominal hollowing	As the subject hollows the abdomen, ask them to count out loud to ten. Breath holding then becomes obvious to them

Fig. 44 *Common mistakes when performing abdominal hollowing actions*

MULTIFIDUS SETTING

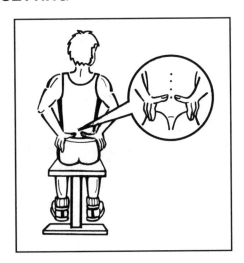

■ Starting position
Sit at the edge of a stool with your knees and feet shoulder width apart. Place your thumbs in the small of your back just above waistband level. They should be placed to the side of the bones of your spine (spinous processes), and pressed in to the skin gently.

■ Action
Gently draw your tummy in (hollowing) and at the same time, gently press your deep back muscles against your thumbs.

■ Points to note
The action must be restricted to your deep back muscles. You should not lean or push yourself back, nor hollow or flatten your spine substantially. Only a small local movement of the spinal bones should be felt. Because your knees are apart, you begin with your lower spine slightly hollow. As the multifidus muscle contracts, it will gently deepen the lumbar curve to bring you back towards the neutral back position.

■ Training tip
Most people find it difficult to feel this muscle contract, so persevere. It is often what you don't feel which is important. As you tighten your back muscles you should not feel the large columns of muscle at either side of the spine tighten (these are the erector spinae muscles). Try to focus the muscle action to within 2 cm (1 in.) of the centre of the back. It is helpful to perform a pelvic floor contraction at the same time as tightening the multifidus.

PELVIC-FLOOR CONTRACTIONS

■ Starting position
Lie on the floor with the knees and feet slightly apart. Relax your buttock muscles (gluteals) and the muscles which pull your legs together (adductors).

■ Action
Slowly tighten (draw up) the muscles around your back passage (anus). Hold this feeling and try to take it forward to tighten the muscles around the vagina (female) or to lift the penis slightly (male). The feeling should be as though you are trying to stop yourself passing water. Hold for a count of 5 (breathing normally) and then release.

■ Points to note
This action is just as important in the male as it is in the female, because the pelvic-floor muscles work with the deep corset muscles in core stability. In addition, the pelvic-floor muscles work to prevent 'dribbling' of urine (incontinence) and to help maintain an erection in the male. Try to perform the action without tensing the gluteal or adductor muscles

■ Training tip
Although the action should *feel* the same as trying to stop the passage of urine, do not perform the action while actually passing urine. This is because this action may interfere with the natural reflexes which control the bladder and can make it hard to pass urine in the normal way.

LEVEL ONE

HEEL SLIDE •

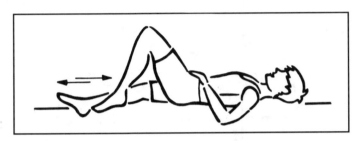

■ Starting position
Begin lying on the floor on your back. Your feet and knees should be 10–15 cm (4–6 in.) apart. Put your hands on your tummy, with the heel of the hand over your pelvic bones. Place the heel of each foot on a shiny piece of paper on a carpet, or a soft cloth on a hard wooden floor.

■ Action
Perform the abdominal hollowing action and hold the abdomen tight. Feel the muscles tense beneath your fingers. Continue to breathe normally throughout the exercise. Slide one leg out straight while holding your tummy tight. As soon as the heel of your hand feels your pelvis begin to tip, slide the leg back in again.

■ Points to note
The aim of this exercise is to build up the ability of the abdominal muscles to hold the pelvis firm. The action of the leg muscles is therefore secondary to that of the abdominals.

■ Training tip
The weight of your leg should be taken by the floor throughout the movement. Do not lift your heel up from the ground. The action is to *slide*, not to lift.

LEG SHORTENING, LYING ● ● ● ● ● ● ● ● ● ● ● ● ● ● ● ● ● ●

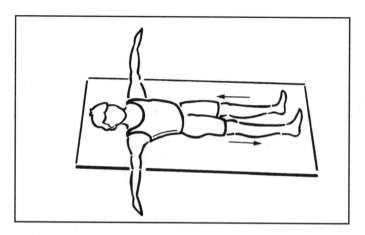

■ Starting position
Begin lying on the floor on your back with your feet 20 cm (8 in.) apart. Place your arms out sideways in a 'T' shape.

■ Action
Tip your pelvis from side to side ('hitching the hip') to shorten and then lengthen each leg.

■ Points to note
The leg must remain perfectly straight to focus the movement on the pelvis, and through this on to the lower spine.

■ Training tip
Flex your foot, and lead the movement with your heel.

SIDE LYING, SPINE LENGTHENING •••••••••••••••

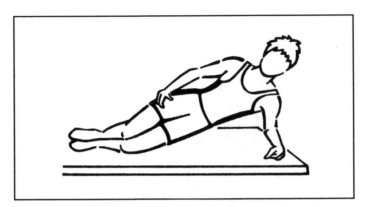

■ Starting position
Lie on your side with your knees together and slightly bent.
Prop yourself up on one elbow so that your back is gently
curved.

■ Action
Tighten (hollow) your tummy and lift the lower side of the trunk
upwards so that you straighten your spine. Hold the position for
5 seconds and then lower.

■ Points to note
Hollowing tightens the muscles at the front and sides of your
tummy, while this exercise tightens the side muscles still further.
The result is that you feel improved muscle tone around the
whole of your waist.

■ Training tip
Do not lift the underneath hip, simply allow it to rock gently on
the floor as you straighten the spine.

ABDOMINAL HOLLOWING AND LEG STRAIGHTENING • • • •

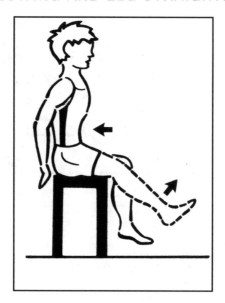

■ Starting position
Sit on a chair or stool with your feet *off* the ground. Tighten (hollow) your abdomen and sit up straight, lengthening your spine.

■ Action
Keep your tummy muscles tight (hollow) and gradually straighten one leg, maintaining your normal back alignment.

■ Points to note
When you straighten one leg, tension in the hamstring muscles at the back of the leg will pull on your sitting bone (ishial tuberosity) and try to tilt your pelvis backwards, rounding your lower back. Make sure that you maintain your alignment and prevent this from happening.

■ Training tip
If your training partner places their hand about 1–2 cm (½ in.) behind the small of your back, they will be able to monitor the lumbar hollow (lordosis) and tell you if your alignment is being lost.

LEG LOWERING, SUPINE • • • • • • • • • • • • • • • • • • •

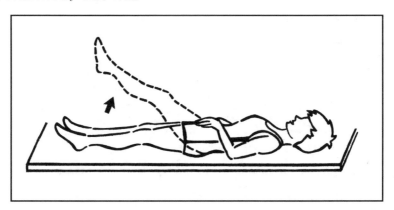

■ Starting position
Lie on the floor with your feet comfortably apart. Place your finger tips on either side of your tummy below the level of your tummy button.

■ Action
Tighten (hollow) your abdomen and hold it tight throughout the exercise. Raise one leg (keeping it straight) to a count of 1, to 45° above the horizontal. Pause in this position and then lower the raised leg back to the floor to a count of 5. Rest in the lying position for 2 seconds and then repeat with the other leg.

■ Points to note
On no account should both legs move together. Do not lift the second leg until the first is back on the floor and you have rested for 2 seconds. If you find the exercise too hard, bend both knees and lift the leg with the knee bent. This will shorten the leg lever and make the exercise easier.

■ Training tip
Monitor the position of your tummy with your fingertips. If you feel your tummy bulging ('ballooning') rather than staying flat, stop the exercise.

TRUNK CURL SEQUENCE ● ● ● ● ● ● ● ● ● ● ● ● ● ● ● ● ● ● ●

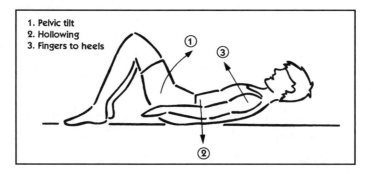

1. Pelvic tilt
2. Hollowing
3. Fingers to heels

■ Starting position
Begin lying on your back with your knees bent. Your feet should be shoulder width apart.

■ Action
Perform the pelvic tilt and flatten your back on to the floor. Next, perform the abdominal hollowing action, pulling your tummy button in. Finally, reach forwards with your fingers towards your heels so that your trunk bends and your shoulders lift away from the floor.

■ Points to note
The action of this exercise is to *bend the trunk*, not to sit up. The bottom part of the shoulder blades should stay in contact with the ground throughout the movement. As you perform the abdominal hollowing action, breathe out. Breathe in as you release the movement.

■ Training tip
Reaching forwards (along the ground) towards the heels, rather than upwards for the knees, encourages the correct trunk bending action.

ABDOMINAL HOLLOWING WITH GLUTEAL BRACE • • • • • •

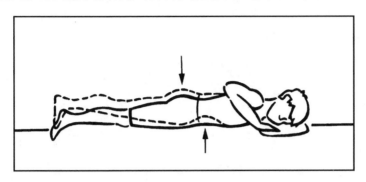

■ Starting position
Begin lying on your front on the floor. Tuck your feet under so your toes are flexed. Place a folded towel beneath your forehead for comfort.

■ Action
Perform the abdominal hollowing action by pulling your tummy in tight, focusing your attention on your tummy button. At the same time, tighten your buttocks and brace your legs out straight.

■ Points to note
You must maintain the neutral position of your spine throughout the action. Make sure you don't tilt your pelvis forwards or backwards.

■ Training tip
Tighten your tummy first, and then grip your buttocks together. Once you have mastered the individual actions, try performing both at the same time.

'X' TONE ●

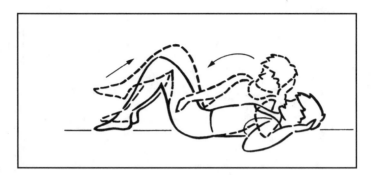

■ Starting position
Begin lying on the floor on your back with your knees bent, feet flat. Your knees and feet should be about 20–30 cm (8–12 in.) apart.

■ Action
Reach past the outside of your right knee with your left hand. At the same time, lift your right foot off the ground and pull the right side of your pelvis towards you. Pause, and then reverse the action, reaching to the left.

■ Points to note
The aim of this exercise is to tone the oblique abdominals. To achieve this, the lower part of the trunk must take part in the action, so the hip pull is essential to the exercise.

■ Training tip
To emphasise the hip pull action, initially ask someone to press on to your hip as you pull. This will make isolating the action easier. *Remember to lift only one hip at a time!*

LEVEL TWO

LEG LOWERING FROM CRUNCH POSITION ● ● ● ● ● ● ● ● ● ● ●

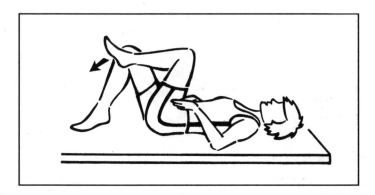

■ Starting position
Lie on the floor and draw your knees up to rest above your hips – feet off the floor – moving one knee at a time. Place your fingertips on either side of your lower abdomen below your tummy button.

■ Action
Tighten your tummy muscles to hollow your abdomen, and maintain this muscle contraction throughout the exercise. Slowly lower one leg, keeping it bent, until your foot touches the floor. Raise the leg again and, when it is in the starting position again, begin to lower the other leg.

■ Points to note
The foot should be lowered directly downwards, keeping it in close to the buttocks. Do not allow the leg to straighten even slightly, as this will place excessive stress on the lower back.

■ Training tip
Monitor the position of your tummy and pelvis with your fingertips. If you feel your tummy bulging ('ballooning') rather than staying flat, or if you feel your pelvis move, stop the exercise.

PELVIC RAISE (1) •

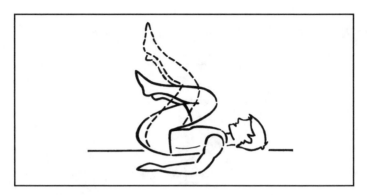

■ Starting position
Begin lying on the floor on your back. Your arms should rest on the floor by your sides (palms down) making an angle of 45° to your body. Bend your knees and draw them up on to your chest.

■ Action
Bend your spine to lift your tailbone 3 cm (1 in.) off the ground, at the same time pulling your knees upwards towards your shoulders.

■ Points to note
Do not lunge into the movement using the momentum of your legs. The action should be a gentle raising of the lower spine, with the power of the trunk muscles lifting the inactive legs.

■ Training tip
Press down hard with your straight arms on to the floor as you flex your lower spine.

BENCH CRUNCH •

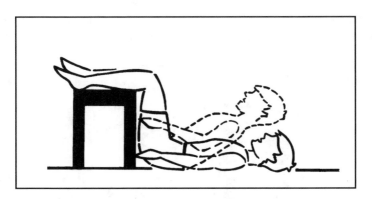

■ Starting position
Begin lying on the floor on your back. Place your calves on a low chair or stool so that your knees and hips are bent to 90°. Your feet and knees should be 20–30 cm (8–12 in.) apart.

■ Action
Sit forwards, as though trying to touch your chest flat on to your thighs.

■ Points to note
This is an advanced exercise and as such you may not be able to lift forwards very far to begin with. Do not speed the movement up in an attempt to sit up further. This will simply increase the momentum of your trunk but will not work the abdominal muscles harder.

■ Training tip
Try to bend your trunk as you begin to sit forwards, to shorten the abdominal muscles.

OBLIQUE BENCH CRUNCH ● ● ● ● ● ● ● ● ● ● ● ● ● ● ● ● ● ●

Do not attempt this exercise until you can comfortably perform ten repetitions of the bench crunch.

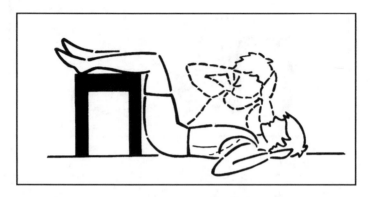

■ Starting position
Begin lying on the floor on your back. Place your calves on a low chair or stool so that your knees and hips are bent to 90°. Your feet and knees should be 20–30 cm (8–12 in.) apart. Fold your arms lightly, keeping your elbows bent to 90°.

■ Action
Sit up, and at the same time reach your right elbow past your left knee. Pause and then repeat the action, reaching with your left elbow past your right knee.

■ Points to note
As with the bench crunch, make sure that the exercise is performed slowly, under control. A rapid action will enable you to sit up further, but only through momentum.

■ Training tip
Exhale hard as you sit up, but rest after each pair of oblique crunches, and breathe normally so you do not get dizzy.

KNEE ROLLING ●

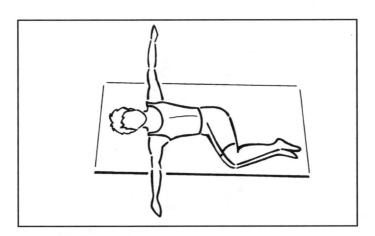

■ Starting position
Lie on your back with your knees bent, feet flat on the floor. Place your arms out sideways in a 'T' shape to aid stability.

■ Action
Perform the abdominal hollowing action, and hold the tummy muscles tight throughout the movement. Allow the knees to slowly lower to one side, forming an angle of about 30° to the vertical. Pull the knees back to the mid-position and then repeat the action.

■ Points to note
Breathe normally throughout the exercise; do not hold your breath. Make sure you keep both hips on the ground as you lower the knees.

■ Training tip
If you cannot lower your knees to the ground, place a cushion on the floor at either side of your hips. Lower your knees on to the cushion rather than right down on to the floor to begin with.

BRIDGING • •

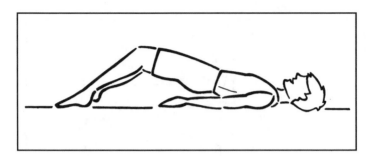

■ Starting position
Begin lying on your back with your knees bent and feet flat on the floor. Your feet should be shoulder width apart. Find your neutral position and maintain this throughout the exercise.

■ Action
Perform the abdominal hollowing action and then tighten your buttock muscles and lift your hips 10 cm (4 in.) from the floor.

■ Points to note
The lower spine must stay in its neutral position, so make sure that you don't lift too high or your spine will arch. Your tummy and upper leg should be in line.

■ Training tip
Allow the squeeze of the buttock muscles to lead the movement and lift you, rather than leading with your stomach.

BRIDGING ON A GYM BALL • • • • • • • • • • • • • • • • • •

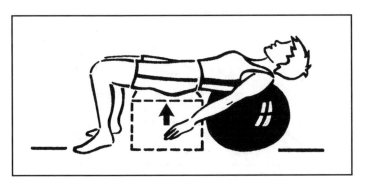

■ Starting position
Lie with your shoulders on a gym ball and your feet shoulder width apart.

■ Action
Tighten (hollow) your tummy and raise your hips from the floor to the horizontal position. Hold this position for 3–5 seconds and then slowly lower.

■ Points to note
You must make sure that you keep your tummy tight throughout the action and avoid allowing your back to hollow excessively.

■ Training tip
If you find it difficult to lift into the position, begin with your hips on a block or low stool and raise from here. The gym ball is an unstable surface and this makes your trunk muscles work harder to maintain your own core stability. However, until you get used to the exercise you can stop the ball from rolling by placing it on a ball ring, available from gym ball suppliers.

SIDE LYING BODY LIFT

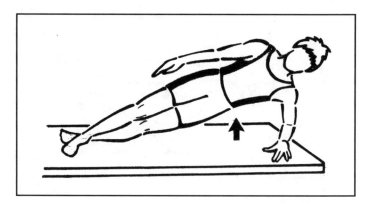

■ Starting position
Begin lying on your side on a gym mat. Place your top foot in front of your bottom foot and keep your legs straight. Prop yourself up on your underneath forearm, and tighten (hollow) your abdomen.

■ Action
Raise your body so that your spine is straight and you are just balanced on your feet and underneath forearm.

■ Points to note
The underneath side trunk muscles (obliques) are working in this exercise together with your deep corset muscles.

■ Training tip
Make sure you broaden your shoulders as you lift so that you don't feel that they are 'bunched up'.

PELVIC RAISE (2) ●

You must be able to perform 5–10 repetitions of pelvic raise (1) before attempting this exercise.

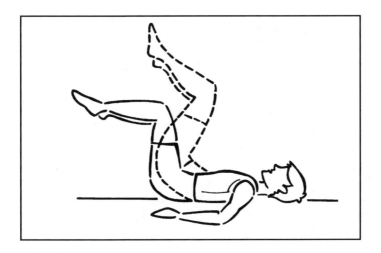

■ Starting position
Begin lying on the floor on your back. Your arms should rest on the floor by your sides (palms down), making an angle of 45° to your body. Bend your knees and hips to 90°.

■ Action
Bend your spine to lift your tailbone 3 cm (1 in.) off the ground, while holding your hips still.

■ Points to note
This exercise works the lower abdominals hard. However, work is taken off these muscles if rapid hip flexion is used to lever the spine off the floor. The hips should stay inactive throughout the movement, with the power of the exercise coming from the lower abdominals only. Keep the knees off the chest.

■ Training tip
Press down hard with your straight arms on to the floor as you flex your lower spine. Begin by lifting the tailbone and then the last spinal bone followed by the next to last.

SIDE BEND IN SIDE LYING ● ● ● ● ● ● ● ● ● ● ● ● ● ● ● ● ● ●

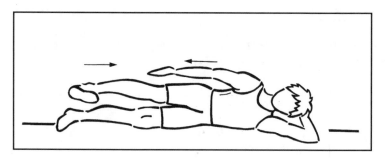

■ Starting position
Begin lying on your side on a mat. Bend your lower arm and leg slightly to improve your stability. Rest your head lightly on your hand for support.

■ Action
Perform a side-bending action so that your lower shoulder lifts from the floor by 2 cm (¾ in.). At the same time, 'hitch' your upper leg so that you shorten it by 2 cm (¾ in.).

■ Points to note
The total side-bend movement is very small, so neither the trunk nor the leg should lift very far.

■ Training tip
Imagine you are 'gathering' the skin at the side of the trunk as your trunk pulls in one direction and your leg in the other.

ROPE CLIMB •

Do not attempt this exercise until you can perform ten repetitions of the trunk curl and bench crunch comfortably.

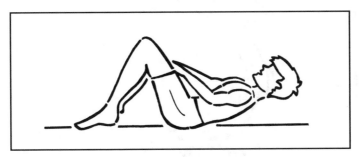

■ Starting position
Begin lying on the floor with your knees bent, arms by your sides. Your feet and knees should be 20–30 cm (8–12 in.) apart.

■ Action
Imagine a line joining your knees, and focus on a point just above the centre of this line. Reach up with your right hand for this point by curling and twisting your trunk. Pause and then allow yourself to sit back down partially. Immediately reach up with the other hand to the same point, and then continue to repeat the action.

■ Points to note
The lower spine should stay on the ground; only the chest and shoulders lift up. Keep the trunk curled throughout the movement so that you maintain tension in the abdominal muscles. Breathe normally throughout the movement; *do not* hold your breath.

■ Training tip
As you reach towards the high point in this movement, grip as though you are pulling on a rope. As you lower down, keep reaching forwards with your arm to maintain the curled position of the trunk.

NEGATIVE CRUNCH ●

Do not attempt this exercise until you can perform ten repetitions of the trunk crunch comfortably.

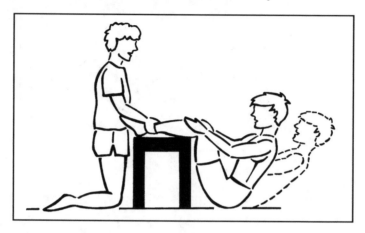

■ Starting position
Begin lying on a mat on your back. Place your calves on a low chair or stool so that your knees and hips are bent to 90°. Your feet and knees should be 20–30 cm (8–12 in.) apart. Fix your feet by hooking them under an object or ask a training partner to hold them firmly.

■ Action
Reach forwards and grip your knees. Pull yourself up using just arm strength until your chest touches your thighs. Flex your trunk so your head touches your knees, and maintain this flexed position throughout the exercise. Slowly lower your upper body back down on to the floor inch by inch, taking a total of 30 seconds to complete the movement.

■ Points to note
Make sure you breathe normally throughout the movement; *do not* hold your breath.

■ Training tip
Make sure your tail touches the floor first, followed by the small of your back, the mid-back, shoulder blades and finally the shoulders themselves.

STRAIGHT LEG ROLL •

Do not attempt this exercise until you can perform ten repetitions of knee rolling comfortably.

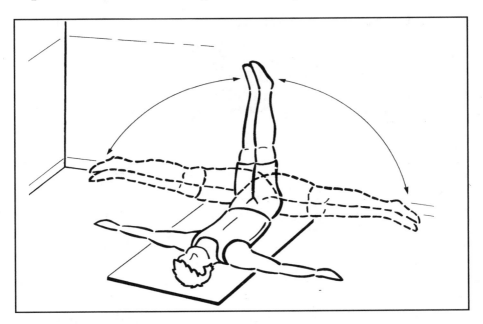

■ Starting position
Lie on the floor with your knees bent. Stretch your arms out to the side in a 'T' shape to aid stability. Draw your knees up on to your chest and then straighten your legs so that your hips, knees and feet are in line.

■ Action
Gradually lower your legs, keeping them straight, sideways on to the floor. Keep the arms and shoulders pressed tightly against the floor for stability.

■ Points to note
The hips remain on the floor as the trunk twists. Make sure the action stays controlled. *Do not* allow the legs to drop rapidly to the floor.

■ Training tip
When you begin the exercise, place two cushions on the floor at either side of your hips. Start the exercise by lowering your legs on to the cushions rather than the floor.

DOUBLE LEG HOLD USING GYM BALL • • • • • • • • • • • •

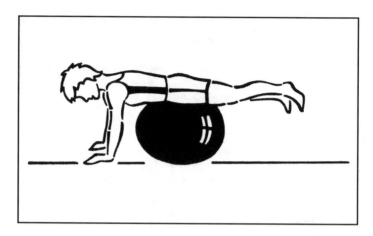

■ Starting position
Begin in the press-up position with your shins on a gym ball. Your hands should be slightly wider than shoulder width apart. Tighten (hollow) your tummy muscles and hold them tight throughout the exercise.

■ Action
Keep your legs straight and horizontal, and walk your hands backwards towards the ball, so the ball moves up your body to your waist. Hold this position for 3–5 seconds and then walk your hands back to the starting position.

■ Points to note
The aim of this exercise is to maintain alignment by tensing the abdomen, buttock, and back muscles. A balanced contraction between these muscle groups is required without one muscle group dominating. It is essential therefore that the body is *in line*; the legs should not be extended above the horizontal and the back should not hollow excessively.

■ Training tip
To begin with, walk the arms towards the ball until the ball rests at knee level. Once this is comfortable, walk the arms further until the ball rests at the hips. Finally, walk the arms so that the ball rests at the waist. In this way the exercise intensity is increased gradually (progressively).

Aʙ FRAME CRUNCH •

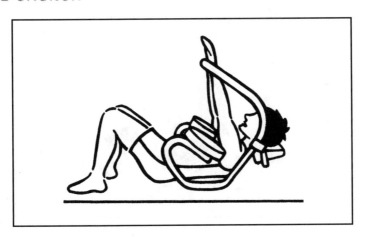

■ Starting position
Begin lying on a mat with your knees bent and slightly apart. Place your hands on the handles of the ab frame and your head on the head-rest. Tighten (hollow) your abdomen.

■ Action
Curl the trunk while resting your head gently on the machine head-rest. Hold the upper position and then slowly lower.

■ Points to note
The aim of the ab frame is to assist the movement and maintain good alignment. Make sure that you keep your head on the head-rest and use only enough hand pressure on the frame to enable you to perform the action smoothly. If you find yourself pushing back hard on to the head-rest, allow your neck and upper spine to bend a little and look through your knees.

■ Training tip
As you get tired, you will need to use more hand pressure on the frame. When this happens, make sure that you keep the movement slow and controlled, avoiding any jerking actions.

AB FRAME REVERSE CRUNCH ● ● ● ● ● ● ● ● ● ● ● ● ● ● ● ● ●

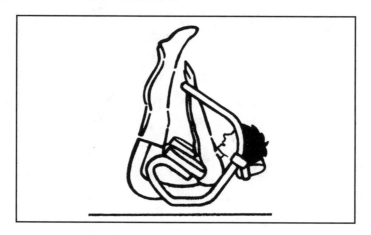

■ Starting position
Lie on the floor with your knees bent. Place your head on the head-rest of the ab frame and hold on to the handle. Tighten (hollow) your tummy, and then lift first one leg to the vertical position, and then the other. Make sure you keep your knee bent as you lift the leg and straighten it only when the knee is above the hip.

■ Action
Keep the upper body still and slowly lift your legs as though you were trying to touch the ceiling with your toes. Hold the upper position for 1–2 seconds and then slowly lower.

■ Points to note
The action is to tilt the pelvis backwards by flattening the back against the floor and then lift the tailbone.

■ Training tip
There is very little movement involved with this exercise. Aim to lift the waistband of your shorts about 2 cm (1 in.) from the floor.

Abdominal Training in Sport and Exercise Classes

The principles which make up the F.L.A.T. programme may be used in sport in two ways. Firstly, the exercises described earlier may be incorporated into a general training programme. This will have the effect of making the trunk section of any training programme far safer and more effective. In addition, because the arms and legs depend on the stability of the trunk as the core against which they push and pull, the function of the limbs may well improve. Finally, the programme can contribute by using the underlying principle of enhanced trunk stability to provide the foundation for movements in all sports actions. The following exercises demonstrate a few examples of how commonly used exercises can be modified using F.L.A.T. principles to improve safety and effectiveness.

WEIGHT TRAINING

We have seen that the neutral position of the spine should be maintained as often as possible to reduce stress acting on the lumbar region. One of the ways of doing this and of stabilising the spine is to practise the abdominal hollowing action. By pulling the abdominal muscles in tightly, the trunk becomes more stable and body alignment is improved. In fig. 44a, the athlete is performing a shoulder press action. The pelvis has tipped forwards and the lumbar curve has become excessive. By tightening the abdominal muscles (*see* fig. 44b), the pelvis will remain level and the lumbar spine is correctly aligned. In addition, the athlete in fig. 44b has widened the base of support and is therefore more stable. The combination of stable spine and stable base makes the exercise far safer.

The same applies to fig. 45. Initially, the athlete performing the arm curl has allowed the pelvis to tip forwards and is dangerously overextending the spine to swing the weight upwards. In fig. 45b, by modifying the exercise using the programme's

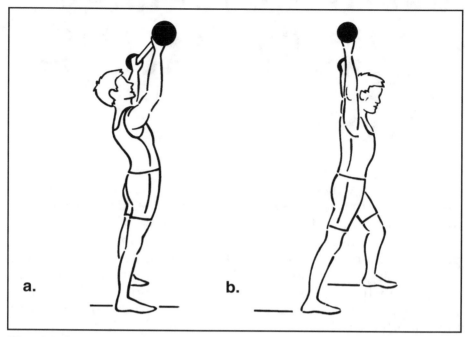

Fig. 44 *Shoulder press: (a) stress on lower spine – unstable position; (b) spine correctly aligned – more stable position*

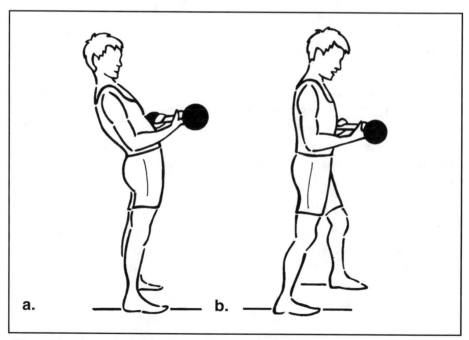

Fig. 45 *Arm curl: (a) back arching, spine dangerously overextended; (b) feet apart, spine aligned, abdominals tight*

principles, the exercise is far safer. Firstly, abdominal hollowing has been used to correct the pelvic tilt and give the athlete a stable trunk to work from. Secondly, the base of support has been widened by placing the feet one in front of the other, and the knees are bent so that the legs, rather than the spine, give the spring to the action.

In fig. 46 the athlete is performing a squat exercise. There are a number of errors in technique here which are making the exercise quite dangerous to the spine. Firstly, the pelvis has tipped right forwards, allowing the abdominal muscles to lengthen and protrude. This increases the lumbar curve and fails to stabilise the spine. In addition, the knees are not bent sufficiently to lower the weight. Instead the athlete has tipped the trunk forwards on the hip and allowed the spine to move forwards of the ideal posture line. The weight has been pulled forwards, and the leverage (measured as the distance between the weight and the posture line) has increased dramatically. By applying the F.L.A.T. principles with regard to spinal stability and posture, the exercise has been modified in fig. 46b. The athlete has corrected his posture by bending the knees more (the ankles are raised on a block). This has lowered the weight while keeping the spine and

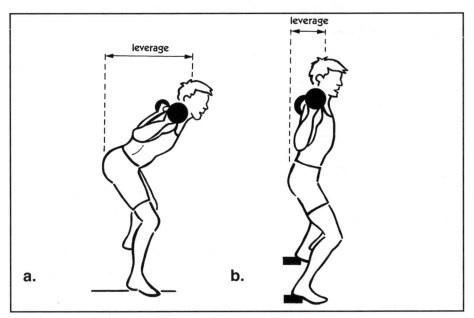

Fig. 46 *Squat exercise: (a) pelvis tipped forwards, increased lumbar curvature, knees not bent, dangerously increased leverage; (b) knees bent more (ankles raised on block), pelvis level, spine more stable*

weight close to the posture line. The pelvis is level and the abdominal muscles have been pulled tight by performing the abdominal hollowing action. The spine is therefore more stable and less likely to be injured through excessive joint movement.

SPECIFIC EXERCISES WITH WEIGHTS • • • • • • • • • • • • •

SIDE BEND

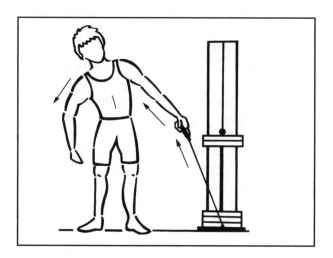

▓ Starting position
Begin standing side-on to a pulley machine. Your feet should be shoulder width apart and facing forwards. Grip the handle of a low pulley unit in your left hand, taking up any slack in the machine cord. Maintain an optimal posture.

▓ Action
Side bend your trunk to the right, reaching down the side of your right leg to try to touch the outside of your knee. Pause and then slowly lower the weight to stand upright again.

▓ Points to note
Make sure that you do not lean forwards or backwards as you perform the side bend. Keep your shoulders and hips square throughout the movement, and do not allow your knees to bend.

▓ Training tip
Focus your attention on the side of your trunk just above the hip. Do not swing the action; bend under control.

KNEE ROLLING

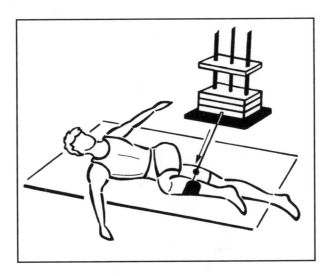

■ Starting position

Begin lying on your back with one knee bent. Attach a sling from a low pulley machine around your bent knee. Place your arms out in a 'T' shape to aid stability.

■ Action

Perform the knee rolling action, lowering your bent knee to the ground away from the pulley. As you do this the weight will lift. Pause and then bring your knee back to the upright position again by lowering the weight.

■ Points to note

The weight must move under control throughout the movement. Do not allow the weight to pull you. Once you have performed ten repetitions to one side, change your position to face the other way and perform ten repetitions to this side.

■ Training tip

If you find the sling from the weight pulley digs into your knee, wrap a towel around your knee beneath the sling before you start.

TRUNK FLEXION FROM HIGH PULLEY

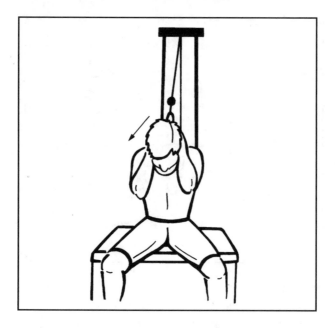

■ Starting position
Begin sitting astride a bench with your hands behind your neck. Grip the handle of a high pulley unit in both hands, behind your neck.

■ Action
Flex your trunk, bending it without leaning forwards to lift the weight. Pause and then lower the weight by straightening your trunk again.

■ Points to note
The action must be one of trunk bending, not bending from the hips.

■ Training tip
Try to imagine you are aiming to touch your nose to your waist, rather than your nose to your knees. The direction of movement must be down, not forwards.

SIDE BEND FROM ABDOMINAL BENCH

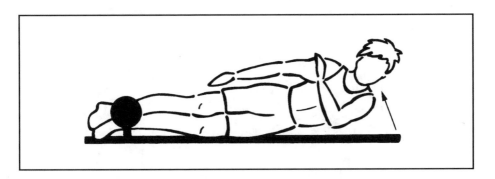

Starting position
Lie on your side on a flat sit-up bench. Hook your feet under the pads, with your upper leg forwards, and lower leg back. Fold your lower arm across your chest and grip your upper shoulder with your hand. Reach along the side of your upper leg with your upper arm.

Action
Perform a side bend action, trying to lift your lower shoulder off the bench. Pause and then slowly lower to the starting position.

Points to note
You may only be able to lift your shoulder by 5–10 cm (2–4 in.). Keep the action strictly to a side bend. Do not lean forwards or backwards.

Training tip
Keep looking forwards as you lift your shoulders, and try to reach your upper hand down towards the side of your upper leg.

SPINAL EXTENSION HOLD

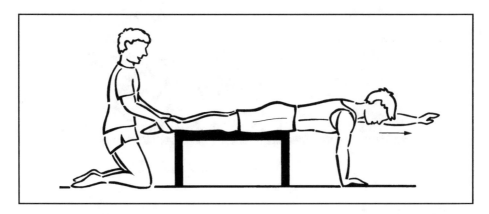

■ Starting position
Begin lying across a gym bench in the press-up position, with a training partner holding your feet down.

■ Action
Perform the abdominal hollowing action to keep your spine in its neutral position. Holding this posture, firstly raise one arm to your side and then both arms. Hold the position and then place your hands back on the ground to rest.

■ Points to note
You must keep your spine straight throughout this exercise; do not allow it to sag. Do not hold your breath; breathe normally.

■ Training tip
Try to reach horizontally with the crown of your head, and 'lengthen the spine' as you perform the action. Build up the time you can hold the movement until you can hold the correct body position for 30 seconds.

EXERCISE TO MUSIC •

The F.L.A.T. principles can be applied to exercise to music (ETM) classes of various types. The aim is to maintain an optimal posture, especially when fatigue sets in towards the end of the class, and to control pelvic angulation when performing other exercises.

During step aerobics, there is a tendency to allow the pelvis to tilt sideways when taking weight on to the stepping foot (*see* fig. 47). This occurs because the hip muscles and abdominal muscles at the side allow the pelvis to sag. As you take your weight on to your foot, stretch the spine and stand tall. Keep your pelvis level but tighten your abdominal muscles, and ensure that your knee is correctly positioned over the centre of your foot.

Many of the trunk exercises used in ETM classes are performed to very high repetitions. As fatigue sets in there is a tendency for quality of exercise technique to suffer. Make sure that you are aware of the angle of your pelvis throughout the exercise bout. Do not allow your spine to extend excessively or maintain a flexed posture for any length of time. Try to keep your pelvis in the neutral position.

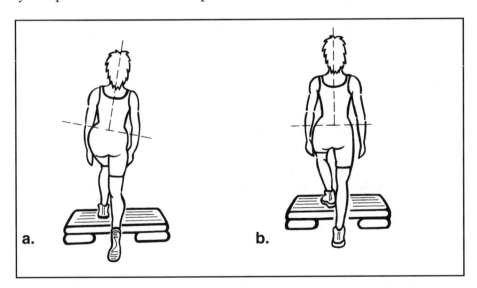

Fig. 47 *Posture during step aerobics: (a) incorrect – pelvis dips, spine leans over, knees have come together; (b) correct – pelvis level, spine lengthened, knees turned out slightly*

Abdominal hollowing is often required to maintain alignment of the spine and pelvis and avoid a 'hollow back' posture (hyper-extension stress). In leg lifting exercises, as the leg reaches its maximum angle of extension, the pelvis will tilt and the lower spine hollow unless the abdominal muscles are first tightened. In the kneeling exercise shown, abdominal hollowing should be performed before the leg is lifted to provide stability to the pelvis and lower spine (*see* fig. 48a). Failure to hollow will increase the apparent range of movement of the hip (*see* fig. 48b) but the new movement is actually only occurring at the spine.

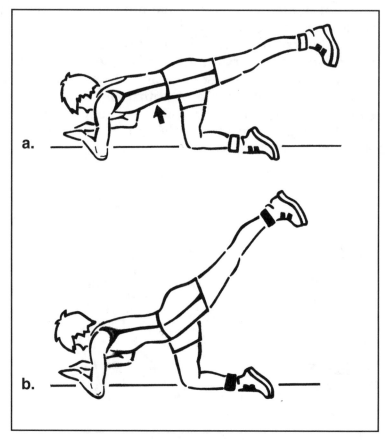

Fig. 48 *Avoiding hyperextension of the lumber spine.*
(a) correct position – abdominals pulled in (hollowed), spine neutral
(b) incorrect position – abdominals lax, pelvis tilted forward and lumber spine hyperextended

SWIMMING

Swimming is traditionally seen as a good exercise after a bout of back pain (*see also* Exercise in Water, pages 141–8). This is because the body is supported by the water and the jarring which often occurs in exercises on hard floors is avoided. However, failure to maintain a neutral position of the spine can still place considerable stress on the back (*see* fig. 49). If breast-stroke is used, for example – a style which allows the head to come high above the water surface and the hips to sink – it places stress on both the neck and lower back. Raising the head above the water is a little like standing and looking up at the ceiling for a long time. The neck vertebrae are compressed, especially those of the upper neck. When this happens the blood flow to the brain is actually reduced and headaches can be the result. Always try to breath out under water when swimming breaststroke so that the head position is lower and the stress to the neck tissues is reduced.

If the hips are allowed to sink, there is more resistance offered by the body. The result is that you have to work harder, and the lower spine is often hyperextended. The abdominal muscles are allowed to relax and lengthen ('ballooning') and the pelvis tips forward. Again the vertebrae are compressed, causing inflammation and pain. The answer is to tighten the abdominal muscles slightly to increase core stability and to swim with the body in a more horizontal position.

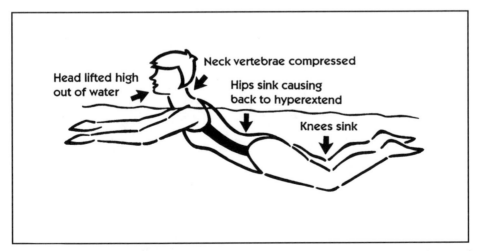

Fig. 49 Incorrect swimming posture

EXERCISING FOR SPEED AND POWER • • • • • • • • • • • •

Many movements in sport are performed rapidly, requiring power and speed. To be specific, the abdominal muscles must be trained to match this power requirement. Because these exercises move the spine quickly, they could be potentially dangerous if performed incorrectly. *To lessen the likelihood of injury, you must be able to perform all the exercises correctly for at least ten repetitions before you attempt the sport-specific training.*

Rapid actions develop speed; rapid actions performed using weight resistance develop power. Each movement should be performed in a specific sequence to build up intensity gradually. Initially the movements should be slow and controlled until the exercise technique is perfected. Later, the speed of movement is gradually built up without resistance. Only when the action can be performed rapidly but in a precise, controlled, fashion should resistance be added. Resistance can increase when the exercises no longer feel challenging. Only light resistances should be used, as heavy weights will slow down the movement and reduce the training effect on power and speed.

MEDICINE BALL CURL-UP

This development of the trunk curl works for explosive power in all the abdominal muscles. It is especially useful for sports such as gymnastics, where lifting the body is performed at speed.

Do not attempt this exercise until you can perform ten repetitions of the trunk curl exercise comfortably.

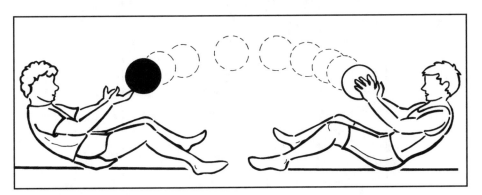

■ Starting position
Begin the exercise lying on your back on a mat with your knees bent, feet flat but not fixed. Your feet and knees should be wide apart – 50 cm (20 in.). Your training partner should be in the same position, with their feet about 15–20 cm (6–8 in.) away from yours. If you increase the distance between you to 35–50 cm (14–20 in.) the exercise becomes even harder.

■ Action
Perform the trunk curl (*see* page 98), and then repeat it using a light, 3 kg (6 lb) medicine ball. As you curl forwards, throw the ball between your knees to your partner, who catches it and throws it back again. Catch the ball in the high position of the exercise and then lower yourself to the floor.

■ Points to note
As for the trunk curl.

■ Training tip
Make sure you keep control of the movement. Do not allow the speed to 'intoxicate you'. Never sacrifice technique for speed, but maintain your alignment throughout the action.

MEDICINE BALL TWIST PASSING

This is useful for building the speed and power of the trunk rotators in combat sports such as judo and wrestling, and also for sports involving rotational movements of the body in space – such as gymnastics, trampolining and board diving.

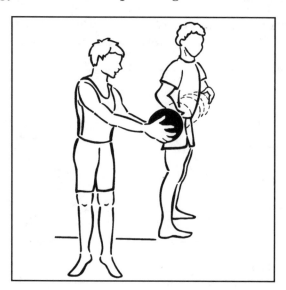

▨ Starting position
Begin standing back-to-back with a training partner, about 25 cm (10 in.) apart. You should both have your feet shoulder width apart, standing tall, holding your abdominal muscles in tight.

▨ Action
Hold a medicine ball in both hands and twist round to the right. Your partner twists to the left, takes the medicine ball and then passes it back to you to their right. The movement should be continuous, like two cog wheels working together.

▨ Points to note
Make sure you do not lean back as the movement speeds up.

▨ Training tips
To increase the overload of the exercise stand further apart and throw the medicine ball using the power of the trunk-twisting action to propel it rather than the arms. Keep the elbows tucked into your sides throughout the movement to reduce the work from the shoulders.

OVERHEAD THROW-IN

This is useful for building control against forces which tend to press the spine backwards into extension – for instance in contact and combat sports. This movement is similar to a soccer throw-in.

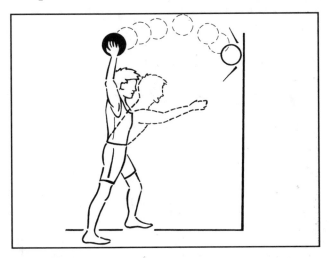

◼ Starting position
Stand facing a wall with one foot in front of the other. Hold a 3 kg (6 lb) medicine ball in both hands.

◼ Action
Lift the ball overhead and extend the spine, keeping the abdominal muscles held in tight. Straighten and then slightly flex the spine to throw the ball at the wall. As the ball bounces off, catch it and control its descent by slightly arching the spine again. Repeat the action.

◼ Points to note
This exercise makes the abdominal muscles work hard to hold the spine stable and prevent it overextending as the ball is thrown and caught. However, excessive movement of the lower spine must be avoided. Be cautious not to overextend the spine when the ball is overhead. The movement should feel comfortable at all times.

◼ Training tip
As the ball bounces off the walls and you catch it, make sure you control it and avoid being pushed into spinal hyperextension. If you find your spine bending too much, throw the ball lower and place your feet further apart.

PUNCHBAG SIDE BEND

Useful for building the trunk side flexors both for power movements (gymnastics and trampolining etc.) and to resist blows (contact and combat sports).

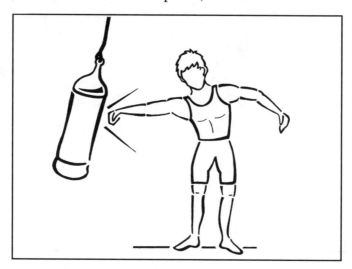

▧ Starting position
Begin the exercise standing side-on to a punchbag. Your feet should be shoulder width apart, and your right arm should be straightened sideways to just touch the punchbag.

▧ Action
Tighten your abdominal muscles and stand tall. Keep your arm straight, and side bend to the right to push the punchbag. As the bag swings back, control your return to an upright body position. Perform ten repetitions and then turn around so that your left arm touches the punch bag and you side bend to the left.

▧ Points to note
Make sure you move with the rhythm of the bag, decelerating it as it swings towards you and accelerating it as you push it away.

▧ Training tip
Begin the exercise slowly, with small range movements. Gradually build up the range of motion and speed individually and then together.

STRETCHING •

We have seen that one of the functions of the programme is to hold the spine stable in its neutral position. We can use this fact to aid us when practising stretching exercises of the muscles which attach to the pelvis. When the stretch is applied, the muscles pull on the pelvis, tending to move it. The F.L.A.T. muscles try to prevent movement by creating a stable base.

When stretching, the stretch should be performed slowly and held for 20–30 seconds. On no account use bouncing movements as these may damage the spine. Breathe out as the stretch is put on to help you relax tight muscles.

HIP FLEXOR STRETCH

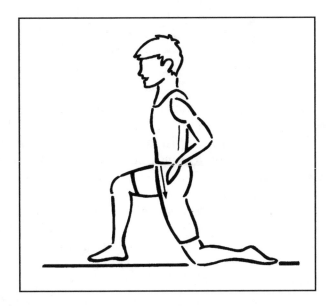

Begin kneeling on one knee with the other leg bent to 90°, foot flat on the floor ('half kneeling'). Place your hand on a chair for support. *Tighten the abdominal muscles* and lunge forwards, causing the back leg to move into extension, and the hip flexor muscles to stretch. If the pelvis remains level, in its neutral position, the back leg will only move to the near vertical. However, if the abdominal muscles relax, the pelvis will tilt and the curve in the lower spine will increase. Now the leg moves back further, not because the hip flexor muscles are being stretched, but because the spine is moving excessively.

HAMSTRING STRETCH, SITTING

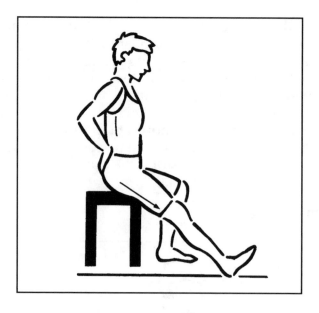

We have seen earlier that the hamstrings are intimately linked to the depth of the curve in the lower back through their direct pull on the pelvis. When sitting, tight hamstrings will tilt the pelvis backwards, rounding the lower back and making back pain more likely. We can take advantage of this fact to exercise the F.L.A.T. muscles and improve sitting posture.

The exercise begins sitting on a low stool, with the knees bent. Sit tall, allowing the lower spine to hollow naturally. Tighten the abdominal muscles using the abdominal hollowing procedure and keep the pelvis level, in the neutral position. Maintaining this correct posture, slowly straighten one leg, feeling the tightness behind the knee. As soon as you feel the pelvis beginning to tilt, you have gone too far. Release the stretch slightly by bending the knee marginally to correct your posture. Maintain the stretch for 20–30 seconds.

ADDUCTOR STRETCH, LYING

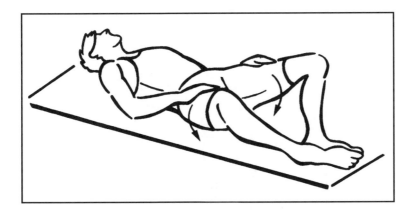

The principles underlying this stretch are similar to those described for the hamstring stretch. If the adductors are tight, when they are stretched they will pull on the pelvis and tilt it, tending to increase the lumbar curve. By using the F.L.A.T. muscles to maintain an optimal posture, we lessen the likelihood of injury.

Begin the adductor stretch by lying on the floor with the knees bent and feet flat. Perform the abdominal hollowing action to fix the pelvis. Keep the feet together, and allow the knees to slowly lower sideways to the floor. As soon as you feel the pelvis tilting, stop the exercise and raise the knees to correct your posture. Hold this new position for 20–30 seconds.

RECTUS FEMORIS STRETCH, STANDING

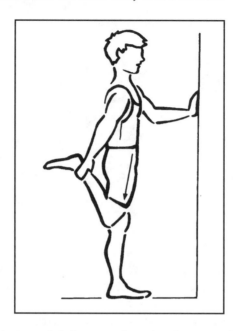

Rectus femoris is a thigh muscle which straightens the knee, but also bends the hip. It is the muscle which is used in kicking, and one which is often damaged by soccer players. Stretching it is important, but performed incorrectly the stretch can place excessive stress on the lower back. By applying the F.L.A.T. principles the exercise is made both safer and far more effective.

Begin standing up straight, holding on to a wall for support. Perform the abdominal hollowing procedure to fix the pelvis. Bend one knee and reach back to take hold of your ankle. Keeping the pelvis level, pull the thigh backwards and at the same time try to bend your knee to touch your heel to your buttock. As soon as you feel your pelvis tilt, release the stretch slightly and correct your posture. Maintain the stretch for 20–30 seconds.

• • • • • • • • • • • • • • • *KEYPOINT* • • • • • • • • • • • • • • • •
Abdominal hollowing is used before the stretch is applied in each exercise. Keep the tummy pulled in tight to protect your lower back.

EXERCISE IN WATER

The principles underlying the F.L.A.T. programme make it suitable for use in water. Water has a number of advantages for exercise involving the spine. The warmth of water is soothing, making it very useful following back pain. In addition, water will support the body, taking some of the bodyweight off the joints and spine and so reducing pain. The muscles responsible for maintaining posture need to work less in water as well because your posture is supported by the water itself.

For the elderly, who may have circulatory problems as well as back pain, water has a further advantage. The pressure variation from the bottom of the pool to the surface actually helps the blood to return to the heart from the legs and so reduces 'tired legs'. Furthermore, the pressure changes created by the depth of the water assist in the reduction in blood pooling (blue veins in the legs) and swelling around the ankles.

PRINCIPLES OF WATER EXERCISE • • • • • • • • • • • • • • •

BUOYANCY

Buoyancy is the degree to which your body will float when it is in water. Your individual buoyancy is determined by your body make-up. Body fat will make you more buoyant, while muscle makes you less. Plump individuals will tend to float, therefore, while those who are skinny are more likely to sink. If you have a large amount of muscle you may find it difficult to keep your legs afloat, so you will need assistance from floats when performing some leg exercises. The depth of the water you are standing in will also affect your buoyancy. The body will float more when it is in deeper water. When the water is waist high, your bodyweight is actually reduced by about 50%. When the water is up to your shoulders, your bodyweight is effectively reduced by 90%, so there is considerably less shock on the joints and spine in deeper water. However, because you float more in deeper water, movement can be harder to control, so be cautious.

•••••••••••••••• **KEYPOINT** ••••••••••••••••
Buoyancy is related to body density. Thinner and more
muscular individuals tend to sink, while those with high body
fat will float.

Buoyancy can be used to support parts of the body, and both to
assist and resist movements. In fig. 49a, the subject is lying flat
in the water, holding on to the siderail of the swimming pool. To
enable them to float they have placed a rubber ring around their
waist, and a smaller ring around their legs. The rings can be
inflated or deflated according to the subject's buoyancy, to allow
the body to float either just beneath the surface of the water or
deeper. This supported lying position enables a selection of
spinal exercises to be performed with the body moving freely in
several directions.

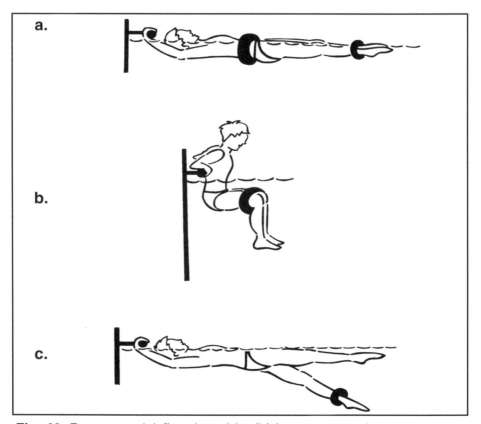

Fig. 49 Buoyancy: (a) flotation aids; (b) buoyancy assistance;
(c) buoyancy resistance

In fig. 48b, buoyancy is being used for assistance. The subject is performing a knee lift movement, but the legs are too heavy to perform the movement correctly. A ring has been placed around the knees to allow the legs to partially float, in effect making them lighter and assisting the upward action of the legs. In fig. 48c, the reverse situation is occurring. The exercise is hip extension, pressing the leg downwards. Now, the buoyancy of the rubber ring tending to lift the leg upwards is acting as a resistance to the downwards movement of the leg.

●●●●●●●●●●●●●●●●● *KEYPOINT* ●●●●●●●●●●●●●●●●●●
Buoyancy can be used to assist or resist a movement, and to support a body part during exercise.

RESISTANCE

Resistance is also provided by the movement of an object through water. The greater the amount of water which has to move, and the faster the object moves, the greater the resistance. Placing the hand side-on (*see* fig. 50a) and moving it slowly through the water provides a certain resistance to the arm muscles performing the movement. If the hand is turned through 90° so that it faces vertically (*see* fig. 50b), it provides considerably more resistance to movement and so the arm muscles must work harder. Speeding up the movement increases the work load still further.

To further boost muscle work we can use apparatus to increase resistance (*see* fig. 50c). Floats placed on their sides and webbed hand gloves are both useful to enhance a water workout.

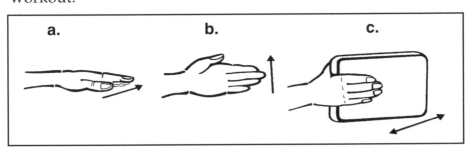

Fig. 50 *Using water resistance: (a) hand parallel to the water surface – little resistance; (b) hand perpendicular to the water surface – greater resistance; (c) using a float standing on its end – maximum resistance*

Because fast movements offer greater resistance, rapid limb movements are useful when working on trunk stability. Standing in deep water and pushing a float rapidly forwards and backwards, for example, will tend to displace the trunk. Tightening the abdominal muscles against this displacement enhances trunk stability.

• • • • • • • • • • • • • • • *KEYPOINT* • • • • • • • • • • • • • • •
Less streamlined objects offer greater water resistance, and can be used to make an exercise harder.

SAFETY CONSIDERATIONS

Obviously water is a dangerous medium to work in, but these dangers can be considerably reduced by taking sensible precautions. Poor swimmers should never practise water exercises in water above waist height, and they must stay close to the poolside at all times. Young children must be continuously supervised, however strong their swimming may appear.

When using apparatus to float, it is easy to become disorientated, and panic. For this reason, always exercise with a partner. When one of you is working, the other should be standing by, offering support and encouragement.

Many accidents occur when moving to and from the pool, so *walk* on wet surfaces, don't run. Also, when getting into and out of the pool, be cautious, and use the steps rather than jumping or diving in, especially with shallow water.

• • • • • • • • • • • • • • • *KEYPOINT* • • • • • • • • • • • • • • •
In water, it's always safety first.

WATER EXERCISES •

TRUNK SIDE BENDING

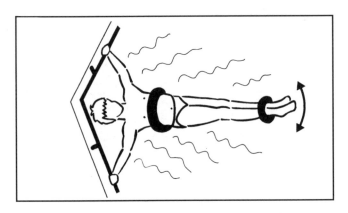

▧ Starting position
Begin the exercise lying on your back in the water, holding on to the siderail of the pool. Choose a wide grip, and keep your arms locked. Ask your training partner to place a rubber ring around your waist, and a smaller (or less inflated) ring around your shins. The rings should be inflated sufficiently to allow your body to float just beneath the surface of the water.

▧ Action
Keep your legs straight and move them from side to side in the water to make your trunk side-flex. Keep the action slow and controlled, and pause as you reach the end point of each sideways movement.

▧ Points to note
Make sure you control the momentum of the movement. Do not allow yourself to be forced into a greater side bending range of motion than you intended.

▧ Training tip
Begin the exercise slowly with small-range movements. Gradually build up the range of motion and speed individually and then together.

LEG SHORTENING AND LENGTHENING

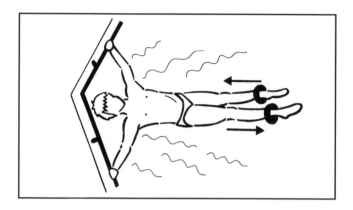

Starting position
As for trunk side bending (*see* page 141). (Some subjects may not require a ring around the waist.)

Action
Keep your body in line, and shorten one leg while lengthening the other, so that your pelvis tilts sideways.

Points to note
Do not allow your spine to flex or extend; isolate the movement to the pelvis.

Training tip
If you find the movement difficult to visualise, have a training partner hold a float at your feet. Watch each foot moving towards and away from the float.

LEG LIFT

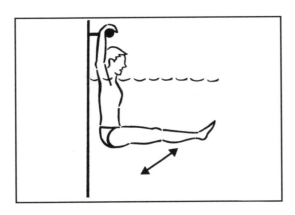

■ Starting position
Hold on to the siderail of the pool above head height. Keep your back flat against the poolside.

■ Action
Lift and lower your legs, keeping them straight, and tighten your abdominal muscles using the abdominal hollowing procedure.

■ Points to note
If you find this movement difficult, place a rubber ring around your legs to assist the lifting motion.

■ Training tip
If the movement seems very easy, perform the action more quickly to increase the resistance.

RESISTED TRUNK ROTATION

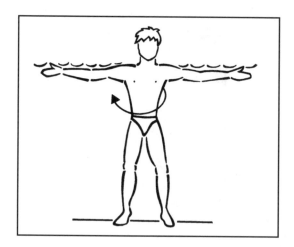

◻ Starting position
Begin the exercise standing in chest deep water within reach of the poolside. Place your feet shoulder width apart and stand tall, pulling your tummy in. Stretch your arms out to the side, keeping them just below the surface of the water. Your hands should be flat at 90° to the surface of the water, fingers together.

◻ Action
Twist your trunk, without bending forwards or backwards.

◻ Points to note
Twist round as far as is comfortable, but do not force the movement.

◻ Training tip
If you find the exercise easy, either wear webbed gloves, or hold a float in each hand positioned at 90° to the water surface to increase resistance. Speeding up the movement will also make the exercise harder, but make sure that you maintain a good posture.

KNEE TWIST

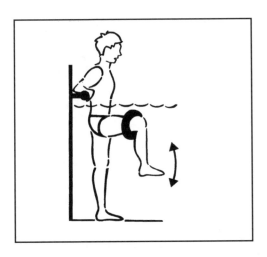

▨ Starting position

Begin the exercise with your back on the poolside, gripping the siderail with outstretched arms. Bend one knee and place a rubber ring around the knee of this leg.

▨ Action

Tighten your abdominal muscles and flatten the small of your back towards the poolside. Keeping the tummy tight, twist the trunk to bring the bent knee across the body and on to the side of the pool. Perform five repetitions to one side, then change legs and perform five repetitions to the other side.

▨ Points to note

Everyone is asymmetrical, and it is common to be able to twist further in one direction than the other.

▨ Training tip

Initially, rather than performing a continuous action, twist, pause, and twist back.

BODY CURL

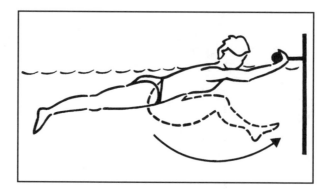

▨ Starting position
Lie on your front, and grip the siderail of the pool.

▨ Action
Bend the legs and trunk to bring your knees towards your chest, and your feet on to the poolside. Pause, and then stretch the body out straight again.

▨ Points to note
The knees begin the movement, followed by the hips and finally the spine. The order is reversed as the legs extend once more.

▨ Training tips
The movement becomes harder if a float is placed around the feet, as buoyancy resists the leg movement under the surface of the water.

USING A FLOATING PLATFORM

The abdominal muscles may also be used for core stability in water by using a movable platform which has a similar effect to the gym ball used earlier in the book. For this you will need a number of flat swimming floats stacked one on top of the other.

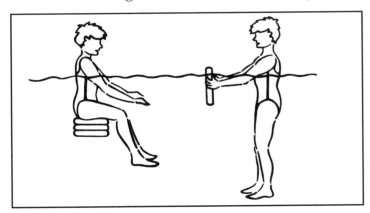

■ Starting position
In shallow water (waist deep or up to lower chest level only) sit on enough floats to allow your body to float in the seated position with the water coming up to the level of your chest.

■ Action
Tighten (hollow) your abdomen and sit up straight. Have your training partner stand in front of you, feet apart. Your partner holds a float vertically and forces the water against you by pushing with their float, while you try to stay sitting upright. You will have to tighten your abdominal muscles harder to do this.

■ Points to note
If you find it difficult to maintain balance while sitting on the platform, move into shallower water so that your feet rest on the bottom. Also use fewer floats to ensure that all of your chest is in the water.

■ Training tip
Once able to maintain your balance, your partner should vary the water current by pushing harder/softer, faster/slower, and from different directions. The aim is to vary the amount of muscle contraction used, to match the changing force of the water being pressed against you.

USING AN AQUATUBE (NOODLE)

Using a smaller seat will also make things harder, and this may be achieved by using an aquatube or noodle.

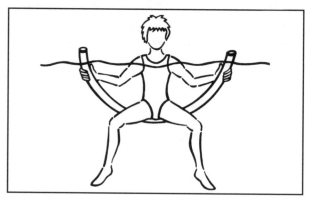

▣ Starting position
With this apparatus, you sit on the tube and grasp the two ends in much the same way as a child sitting on a swing.

▣ Action
A number of actions may then be performed, including pelvic tilting, single- and double-leg raising, trunk rotation and trunk lateral flexion. Placing the aquatube in front of the body and holding on to it gives a point of balance and sufficient flotation to perform single leg movements such as hip scissors (abduction) and trunk movements in general.

▣ Points to note
Different sizes and densities of aquatube are available. Pick one suitable for your body size and weight. Too little buoyancy will mean you sink too low in the water, too much and you will rest too high and won't get the required support from the water.

▣ Training tip
With both the seated float exercise and the aquatube, the abdominal muscles are working hard. Importantly, however, these movements give the additional benefit of varying the intensity of the muscle work (harder or lighter) and making you quickly switch between movements and so change the muscle work rapidly. This rapid change develops the reaction time of the muscle, making it contract and relax more quickly, and is an important part of abdominal training for core stability.

PUTTING IT ALL TOGETHER

We have seen a great many exercises, all designed in some way to enhance core stability. Some are basic, some more advanced. Many are used in combination with stretching or strength training – for example, to achieve core stability as part of an overall training plan. Some are worked in conjunction with postural correction. How do we put it all together to form a coherent abdominal training programme?

Firstly, before embarking on any exercise programme, you must warm up (*see* pages 79–81). Always start with *foundation* movements: for the inexperienced exerciser these may be the only exercises required initially; for the experienced athlete the foundation movements are used as part of a warm-up to 'rehearse' the skills of stability. The key skill is to be able to hollow the abdomen gently, and to maintain this muscle contraction over a period of time. This simple action will enable you to maintain alignment and the 'neutral position' of the lumbar spine (*see* page 10) throughout the exercise programme. Three to five repetitions is all that is required, holding each for 10 seconds while breathing normally.

• • • • • • • • • • • • • • • **KEYPOINT** • • • • • • • • • • • • • • • •
Rehearse abdominal hollowing before you start exercising and maintain the neutral position of the lumbar spine throughout your workout.

Let's now look at some examples of real-life ('functional') situations through some case studies. Remember that these *are* examples and may not exactly match your own requirements. If you have had an injury to the spine you should see a chartered physiotherapist before embarking on core stability training. If you are unsure of your alignment or how to progress your exercise programme, work with a certified personal trainer or exercise professional.

THE OVERWEIGHT INDIVIDUAL • • • • • • • • • • • • • • •

George is a 38-year-old who is about 10 kg (22 lb) overweight. His body fat is 22% and his waist measurement equals his age. A poor diet, too many business lunches and too much alcohol have all taken their toll. He looks and feels 50 and wants to do something about it, but does not know how.

Firstly, diet was the keystone of this programme. He needed to improve the *quality* of his food intake. Less alcohol combined with a reduction in sweet and fatty snack foods started to make an impression. Increasing his intake of fresh fruit and vegetables not only allowed him to loose body fat, but probably dramatically improved his health as well. His diet was combined with regular exercise, and he began with a 10-minute brisk walk each evening and one 20-minute swim each week. This will have increased his metabolic (body 'tick-over') rate for long periods after exercise had finished, and helped to burn calories as well as improving the health of his heart, lungs and circulation. In the first month of his programme his weight came down by 4 kg (9 lb) and his waistline reduced by 2.5 cm (1 in.).

George focused on a single F.L.A.T. exercise, performing abdominal hollowing while standing with his back towards a wall (*see* page 89). Initially he stood looking in a mirror, and also touched his abdominal wall with his fingertips to really appreciate what was happening. By pulling his abdomen away from his waistband and holding the movement while breathing normally, he was able to build the holding time up.

He found the movement very hard to start with. Nothing seemed to happen, but eventually he was able to pull his abdomen from his waistband for 1 or 2 seconds and get the feeling of the exercise. After his first week, practising this movement three times a day, he was able to hold the exercise for 5 seconds. He still found it difficult to keep his rib cage still, but the skill was coming. By week three, George could hold the movement for over 5 seconds and put much less effort into the exercise. He could perform the action without touching his abdomen or looking in a mirror and now used the hollowing action when standing (while shaving in the morning) and also when walking. He found it easier to pull his abdomen away from his waistband for ten steps and then to relax for ten steps while out on his daily 10-minute walk.

After his first month George was ready to move on and began abdominal hollowing in the lying position with his knees bent and from this position the heel slide action was used (*see* page 93). Initially he started with 3 repetitions on each leg and built up to 5 and then 8. His diet was going well and his general exercise was increased. He went to a local gym and began treadmill walking on the flat and then uphill. When his business commitments prevented him from visiting the gym he extended both the length of his walk (15 min) and its intensity (slow to begin, followed by 5 min fast walking and slow to end). In addition, George used a cross-training machine in the gym (5 min) and the rowing machine (5 min). To finish off he performed some supervised light weight training on the seated shoulder press and lateral pull down machine.

> • • • • • • • • • • • • • • *PROGRAMME* • • • • • • • • • • • • • • • •
> Diet to reduce body fat • Cardiopulmonary exercise •
> Abdominal hollowing, standing (using belt) • Abdominal
> hollowing while walking • Heel slide

THE INDIVIDUAL WITH BACK PAIN ° ° ° ° ° ° ° ° ° ° ° ° ° ° ° ●

Julie had lower back pain after the birth of her second child. She is 28 and not overweight, although her body tone is less than it was when she was at college. Her children are aged four and six, and she has back pain especially when bending over to pick up her four-year-old. However, the pain is worse when she sits for a long time and is often so bad than she finds it hard to get to sleep as she cannot easily lie flat.

It turned out Julie had a flatback posture, meaning that the normal curve in her lower back had become flattened out. Her abdominal muscles had poor tone and she had a little 'pot belly' below her umbilicus and, although her general flexibility was quite good, her hamstrings were unusually tight.

Initially Julie was given abdominal hollowing in the kneeling position (*see* page 86) as this was a position in which she had no back pain. She found it difficult to perform the exercise at first – she said that nothing seemed to happen in the tummy! The exercise programme was therefore amended so that it began with pelvic-floor contractions. In conversation Julie admitted that she had not practised these after the birth of her second child and occasionally she 'dribbled' a little urine when she laughed or coughed. When the pelvic-floor contractions were performed, Julie was encouraged to continue the feeling into her lower tummy and feel the umbilicus pulled inwards and upwards. She found this easier when a loose belt was placed around her waist as she was able to feel the muscles pulling away from something. Julie built up the abdominal hollowing to 10 repetitions, holding each for 3 seconds and eventually for 10 seconds, and she practised this twice daily.

To correct her flatback posture Julie did five spinal extension stretches three times a day (*see* page 49). She found this movement quite stiff and sore to begin with but as she persevered the pain gradually eased and the back stretched loose. In addition, Julie was encouraged to practise good back care, limiting the amount of bending that she did and trying whenever possible to bend her knees.

When Julie could perform the abdominal hollowing action easily in the kneeling position, she began to practise the same movement both lying and sitting (*see* page 87 and 88), in each case performing ten repetitions once a day. This led on to leg lowering from supine lying (*see* page 97) and finally leg lowering from a crunch position (*see* page 101). By this time Julie had joined an exercise class and so practised the F.L.A.T. movements three times a week at home. Before each class, however, she still rehearsed abdominal hollowing, and was conscious of her alignment throughout the workout.

To stretch her tight hamstrings, Julie performed abdominal hollowing and leg straightening occasionally during normal activities throughout the day.

• • • • • • • • • • • • • • PROGRAMME • • • • • • • • • • • • • • • •
Pelvic-floor contractions • Abdominal hollowing, kneeling •
Spinal extension stretch • Good back care during the day •
Abdominal hollowing, lying and sitting • Leg lowering from
supine lying • Leg lowering from crunch position •
Abdominal hollowing and leg straightening

Poor stability in an athlete ● ● ● ● ● ● ● ● ● ● ● ● ● ● ● ●

Pooja was a regular at the local gym. She exercised daily, three times per week in the weights room and three aerobic classes, including step and jazz dance. Even at weekends she was active, mountain biking or going for a run. Examination of her trunk showed a classic 'six pack' and a lean honed physique. However, she complained of lower back pain during, and especially the morning after, her weights programme. Two exercises gave her particular problems, the standing hip extension on a 'multi-hip' unit and repeated overhead pressing actions with a light aerobics bar. She reported soreness in the lower back developing gradually and building in intensity until she had to stop the exercise. On close examination of these movements it became obvious that she hyper-extended her spine as she performed both actions. This meant that her pelvis tilted forwards (front part down) and her lower back arched forwards excessively. This is the classic lordotic posture (*see* page 43), and on stretch tests her hip flexor muscles proved tighter than you would expect for a well-trained athlete.

Pooja's problem was not lack of strength – far from it – it was *imbalance*. For her physique and strength, she had very little proportional core stability. As she performed the exercises, her 'corset' muscles (deep abdominals) were unable to hold her spine firmly in its neutral position, and her tight hip flexor muscles were constantly pulling the front of her pelvis down. Her core stability was tested by giving her a heel slide exercise while lying on her back. After only four slow repetitions, her back began to arch away from the ground, whereas an athlete of her calibre should be able to perform 20–30 reps of this movement easily.

Pooja's training programme was modified and all exercises removed which tended to push the spine out of alignment. This included all overhead pressing actions and any hip extension movement. She spent the time saved by deleting these exercises on core stability training. The aim was to enhance core stability, but in addition (and in many ways more importantly) to improve her appreciation of alignment as well by being able to recognise when her spine began to move away from its neutral position. She began with hollowing in the sitting and standing positions (*see* pages 88–9) and was able to learn these actions quickly as her body awareness was excellent from the amount of time she had been exercising. She quickly moved up to leg lowering from a crunch position (*see* page 101) and then progressed to the side lying body lift and the spinal extension hold (*see* pages 108 and 124). In each case the precision of the movement was emphasised and Pooja was encouraged to perform the actions slowly, building up holding time (muscle endurance) to 30–45 seconds.

To retrain her neutral position recognition, Pooja performed pelvic tilting in lying, standing and sitting positions (*see* pages 83 and 85). In each case she was required to move back into the neutral position without looking in the mirror, and with her eyes closed. This type of activity develops 'joint sense' – that is, the ability to recognise the position of a body part by feeling the movement rather than looking at it. This would be important in Pooja's general workout where she would be focusing on the moving weight rather than her mid-body. Pooja also began practising hip flexor stretching exercises kneeling on one knee (*see* page 44), performing the movement slowly and maintaining her neutral spine position throughout the movement.

Finally, Pooja performed her normal gym workout with minimal weight resistance, focusing instead on alignment and maintaining the neutral position with her newly developed core stability. Only when she was able to do this was she allowed to increase her weights or the speed at which she practised her gym programme.

●●●●●●●●●●●●●●●**PROGRAMME** ●●●●●●●●●●●●●●●●
Modified gym programme to remove stressful exercises ●
Abdominal hollowing, standing and sitting ● Leg lowering from a crunch position ● Side lying body lift ● Spinal extension hold ● Pelvic tilting activities ● Hip flexor stretching ● Alignment recognition and practice

---

Abdominal muscle research

The F.L.A.T. method is based on modern training methods developed for physiotherapy and gradually filtered down to the general public. Because discoveries are being made constantly, our knowledge must continually be updated. By looking at some of the research into abdominal training we can see at first hand how the developments begin and how they will affect our normal training programmes.

Which muscles work

Researchers in Brazil[1] looked at twelve different abdominal exercises to distinguish between the work done by the abdominal muscles themselves and that done by the hip flexor muscles – in particular the rectus femoris, which is the large 'kicking muscle' on the front of the thigh. They compared the upper and lower portions of the rectus abdominis muscle of the abdomen in twenty physical education students, and showed that, while leg lifting activities reduced the work on the upper rectus and emphasised the work on the lower portion of the muscle, bending the knees had little effect on the amount of work that the two portions of the muscle performed. Leg lift exercises produced the hardest workloads for the rectus femoris muscle, while curl-up actions produced the lowest. Fixing the feet increased the activity of the rectus femoris still further.

> • • • • • • • • • • • • • • • *KEYPOINT* • • • • • • • • • • • • • • • • • •
> Sit-up type actions emphasise the upper portion of the rectus abdominis, while leg lift movements emphasise the lower portion. Fixing the feet will increase the work on the hip flexor muscles without any real advantage to the abdominal muscles.

Researchers in Australia[2] have looked closely at the difference between the deep muscle corset (the transversus abdominis and multifidus muscles and the internal obliques) and the surface muscles (rectus abdominis, in the centre of the abdomen) and external obliques (at the side). When 'hollowing' the abdomen (*see* fig. 10) as in the F.L.A.T. programme, the internal oblique muscles work harder than the rectus muscle in most people. However, in people who have suffered long standing lower back pain, the internal obliques work less and the rectus works more to try to compensate so that, as well as being weak, an imbalance is created between the two muscles (*see* fig. 51). In order to correct this imbalance, therefore, we must increase the work of the internal oblique muscles, and reduce the work of the rectus. Strengthening both muscles will leave them stronger, but still out of balance.

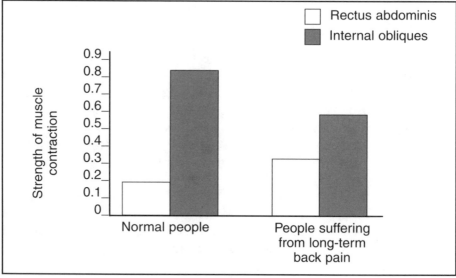

Fig. 51 *Abdominal muscle action in lower back pain*

It is also vital to distinguish between the deep muscles and those on the surface during training. The same researchers[3] looked at a ten-week programme using 15 minutes of core stability exercises (especially abdominal hollowing) daily and compared this to a gym-based programme involving trunk curls and weights. Over the training programme, those using core stability exercises showed a dramatic increase in the activity of the internal oblique muscles but little change in the rectus.

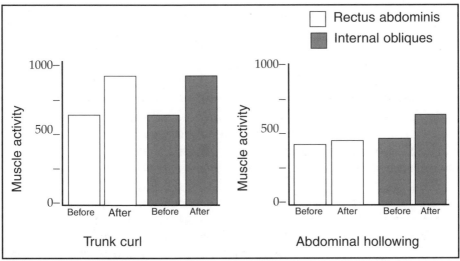

Fig. 52 *Abdominal muscle usage with different types of training*

Those on the gym-based programme, however, showed an improvement in both rectus and internal oblique activity. Although in this case the muscles were stronger after the more traditional gym-based programme, the imbalance between the two sets of muscles still remained (*see* fig. 52).

●●●●●●●●●●●●●●● *KEYPOINT* ●●●●●●●●●●●●●●●●
A muscle imbalance exists in people with back pain whereby the deep (corset) muscles are not used enough and the surface (cosmetic) muscles are used too much. To correct this imbalance, core stability exercises rather than normal gym-based programmes are required.

Physiotherapists at King's College, London[4], looked at the best method to work the transversus muscle (*see* fig 10). They took twenty people and, using the kneeling position, gave half abdominal hollowing on its own, and the other half abdominal hollowing with pelvic-floor contraction. After six weeks the physios then looked at the thickness of the transversus muscle using ultrasound scanning. Abdominal hollowing by itself increased the thickness of the transversus by 49.7% while abdominal hollowing with additional pelvic-floor contraction increased the muscle thickness by 65.8%, a significantly higher score.

This study clearly shows the importance of linking the hollowing action to its normal function in the body. We have seen that hollowing works as part of the abdominal balloon mechanism (*see* page 18) whereby the abdomen can be viewed as a cylinder with the deep muscle corset being the walls and the pelvic-floor muscles the base. Working both muscles at the same time is more effective than simply working one muscle in isolation because the body already recognises the coordination of the muscles pulling together to increase the pressure within the abdominal balloon.

• • • • • • • • • • • • • • • **KEYPOINT** • • • • • • • • • • • • • • • • •
Working the pelvic-floor muscles with the deep muscle corset is an effective method to re-learn core stability.

STRESS ON THE SPINE •

When performing a sit-up-type activity, poorly trained people often allow the lower spine (lumbar region) to hollow excessively, a posture that greatly stresses the spine. This increased lumbar hollow, or 'lordosis', occurs because the abdominal muscles may be too weak to stabilise the spine or the person may simply not be using the muscles correctly. Researchers in Japan[5] looked at the effect of both muscle tensing, and head and neck position, when performing abdominal exercises. They found that sit-up-type actions which involved bending (flexing) the neck and drawing the chin in towards the chest combined with abdominal stabilisation through 'pulling the abdomen in' produced the best results in terms of muscle work. They also x-rayed the spine and showed that pulling the chin in and tightening (stabilising) the abdomen produced the least hollow back and therefore the safest exercise for the lumbar spine.

Researchers at the University of Iowa in America looked at curl exercises and a leg lowering task to determine the effect that a posterior pelvic tilt (pulling the abdomen tight and flattening the back) would have on the abdominal muscles.[6] They looked at the electrical activity of the rectus abdominis, and internal and external obliques in 15 people while they performed either a trunk curl or double straight leg lowering exercise. When people performed the exercises in a neutral position, the rectus abdominis muscle and external obliques dominated the action with little work on the internal obliques. However, when a posterior pelvic tilt was maintained throughout the action, the activity of the rectus was reduced and that of the external and internal obliques significantly increased.

• • • • • • • • • • • • • • • • • **KEYPOINT** • • • • • • • • • • • • • • • • •
Drawing the tummy in (stabilising) and tucking the chin in when performing abdominal exercises helps to prevent the spine from curving inwards excessively and acts to protect the spine. To prevent excessive curvature in the lower back, posteriorly tilt the pelvis (so that you flatten your back).

Researchers from Sweden[7] looked at the effect of abdominal training on intra-abdominal pressure in both healthy people and those with a history of lower back pain. They gave each a series of bent knee curl-ups to do while holding their breath – two sets of ten curl-ups daily over five weeks, during which time both the holding time and resistance of the exercise were gradually increased. The strength of the abdominal muscles increased but the intra-abdominal pressure did not, so the authors concluded that the people could not make functional use of their increased strength because the pattern of movement in training was different from that during lifting.

Scientists from the Department of Neuroscience at the Karolinska Institute in Stockholm, Sweden,[8] looked at the effect of a ten-week specific abdominal strength programme which targeted resisted trunk rotations. Rotation strength increased by nearly 30% after training, and the rate of intra-abdominal pressure development during jumping activities and trunk pushing actions also increased. They therefore concluded that an increase in strength of the trunk rotator muscles with training also increased the rate of intra-abdominal pressure development during functional – in other words, real-life – situations.

• • • • • • • • • • • • • • • • **KEYPOINT** • • • • • • • • • • • • • • • • •
To increase the power of the 'abdominal balloon', the deep muscle corset must be used. Exercises which fail to train these muscles may increase strength and fitness, but will not significantly improve core stability.

ABDOMINAL TRAINING AND APPEARANCE • • • • • • • • • •

Individuals often begin a gym programme with the sole intension of flattening the tummy or 'toning and trimming' the waist. Many researchers have looked at the ability of abdominal training to alter appearance in this way and their findings can be used to guide us to better exercise programmes.

Researchers at the University of Massachusetts[9] looked at the effect of sit-up exercises on the amount of fat around the waist. To assess 'fatness', they used body girth measurements using a tape measure, skin folds measurements, and total fat content using a special machine to detect the amount of fatty tissue in the body. Initially the people in this study undertook an average of 140 sit-ups each day in the first week, and increased this to 336 sit-ups per day by the end of the 27-day training period. The scientists found that there was no real change in any of the fatness measures by the end of the programme. The people were certainly stronger and able to perform a greater number of sit-ups, so muscle training had definitely taken place. However, this training did not include a reduction in body fatness, because this type of training tones and strengthens the muscles. To reduce body fat we need a combination of diet and aerobic (fat burning) exercise such as cycling, jogging or swimming because it increases the 'tick over' of the body (measured as heart rate) for a prolonged period and so burns energy in the form of Calories and ultimately fat.

Maintaining the theme of body appearance, at the University of Norfolk in the US, physical therapy researchers looked at the relationships between lumbar lordosis (low back hollow), pelvic tilt and abdominal muscle performance[10]. We know that lax abdominal muscles can lead to an increased lordosis, and is commonly seen, for example, in obesity and after pregnancy (*see* pages 25–6). However, is there a link between muscle strength and this type of posture? In other words, if your abdominal muscles are stronger, do you have a better posture?

These researchers took 31 physical therapy students and measured their lumbar lordosis and pelvic tilt angle. They then assessed the strength of the abdominal muscles, emphasising the lower (infra-umbilical) part of the rectus abdominis muscle by using a leg lowering task. The students lay on a gym bench, holding on to it above their heads for stability, and were then helped to lift their legs to a vertical position. They then lowered their legs on their own taking 10 seconds to do so, being instructed to keep their backs flat against the bench. As soon as their back began to lift from the bench, the exercise was stopped and the leg angle at which this happened was noted.

The researchers found that there was no relationship between abdominal muscle performance and pelvic tilt or lordosis. Why? The answer is that the abdominal muscles are largely relaxed in normal standing, only becoming active if the trunk is moved. In relaxed standing, it is the length of the abdominal muscles rather than their strength which is important, and when we stand in this fashion the muscles support us, not by contracting, but simply through elasticity. With obesity, over a period of time, the muscles sag and become overstretched, and it is this lengthening which is important from the point of view of relaxed posture.

Two physiotherapists from the University of Queensland in Australia[11] took up this idea and looked at the length of the muscles around the abdomen and the relationship with pelvic angle (pelvic tilt). They looked at 103 adolescent women using a specially designed pelvic angulation measuring device and found that the lengths of the abdominal muscles, the hamstrings and the erector spinae were highly related to lumbar lordosis and could actually be used to predict the depth of the lordosis likely to be found in a given person. This is precisely what is described on page 43, where the balance between the pull of the muscles around the pelvis is discussed. To change posture with exercise, it seems likely that a combination of diet/weight loss with muscle balancing exercise is needed. To change pelvic tilt in obesity, we must reduce body fat, stretch the shortened hamstring muscles and shorten the lengthened abdominal muscles. This is achieved by a combination of deep muscle corset exercise together with the modified trunk curl movement shown on page 98.

• • • • • • • • • • • • • • • • **KEYPOINT** • • • • • • • • • • • • • • • • •
To reduce your waistline you need a combination of diet and regular aerobic exercise. To change your posture you need muscle balancing, rather than pure strength training.

REFERENCES

1. Guimaraes, A. C., Vaz, M. A., De Campos, M. I., Marantes, R. (1991), 'The contribution of the rectus abdominis and rectus femoris in twelve selected abdominal exercises: an electromyographic study', *Journal of Sports Medicine and Physical Fitness*, vol. 31:2, pp. 222–30.
2. O'Sullivan, P. B., Twomey, L. T., and Allison, G. T. (1997), 'Evaluation of specific stabilizing exercise in the treatment of chronic low back pain with radiologic diagnosis of spondylolysis or spondylo-listhesis', *Spine*, vol. 22:7, pp. 2959–67.
3. O'Sullivan, P. B., Twomey, L. T., and Allison, G. T. (1998), 'Altered abdominal recruitment in patients with chronic back pain following a specific exercise intervention', *Journal of Orthopedic and Sports Physical Therapy*, vol. 27, pp. 114–24.
4. Critchley, D. J. (2000), 'Instructing pelvic floor contraction increases transversus adbominis activation in low abdominal hollowing', *Proceedings of the Chartered Society of Physiotherapy Congress* (Birmingham, UK) p. 22.
5. Shirado, O., Ito, T., Kaneda, K. and Strax, T. E. (1995), 'Electro-myographic analysis of four techniques for isometric trunk muscle exercises', *Archives of Physical Medicine and Rehabilitation*, vol. 76:3, pp. 225–9.
6. Shields, R. K., Heiss, D. G. (1997), 'An electromyographic comparison of abdominal muscle synergies during curl and double straight leg lowering exercises with control of the pelvic position', *Spine*, vol. 22:16, pp. 1873–9.
7. Hemborg, B., Moritz, S. and Hamberg, J. (1985), 'Intra-abdominal pressure and trunk muscle activity during lifting – effect of abdominal muscle training in chronic low back patients', *Scandinavian Journal of Rehabilitation Medicine*, vol. 17, pp. 15–24.
8. Cresswell, A. G., Blake, P. L., and Thorstensson, A. (1994), 'The effect of an abdominal muscle training program on intra-abdominal pressure', *Scandinavian Journal of Rehabilitation Medicine*, vol. 26:2, pp. 79–86.
9. Katch, F. I. (1984), 'Effects of sit-up exercise training on adipose cell size and adiposity', *Research Quarterly for Exercise and Sports*, vol. 55, p. 242.
10. Walker, M. L., Rothstein, J. M., Finvcane, S. O. and Lamb, R. L. (1987), 'Relationships between lumbar lordosis, pelvic tilt and abdominal muscle performance', *Physical Therapy*, vol. 67:4, pp. 512–16.
11. Toppenberg, R. M., and Bullock, M. I. (1986), 'The interrelation of spinal curves, pelvic tilt and muscle lengths in the adolescent female', *Australian Journal of Physiotherapy*, vol. 32:1, pp. 6–12.

INDEX

Page numbers in italics refer to illustrations or diagrams; those in bold type refer to the instructions for specific exercises.